Taekwondo
A TECHNICAL MANUAL

Taekwondo
A TECHNICAL MANUAL

Master Gilles R. Savoie

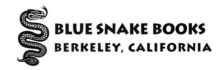
BLUE SNAKE BOOKS
BERKELEY, CALIFORNIA

Published by Blue Snake Books

Blue Snake Books' publications are distributed by

North Atlantic Books
P.O. Box 12327
Berkeley, California 94712

All photos by Gilles R. Savoie

Cover and book design by Brigit Levesque and Sandra Martel

Printed in Canada

Taekwondo: A Technical Manual is sponsored by the Society for the Study of Native Arts and Sciences, a nonprofit educational corporation whose goals are to develop an educational and cross-cultural perspective linking various scientific, social, and artistic fields; to nurture a holistic view of arts, sciences, humanities, and healing; and to publish and distribute literature on the relationship of mind, body, and nature.

North Atlantic Books' publications are available through most bookstores. For further information, call 800-733-3000 or visit our Web sites at www.northatlanticbooks.com. and www.bluesnakebooks.com.

Library of Congress Cataloging-in-Publication Data

Savoie, Gilles R.
Taekwondo : a technical manual / Master Gilles R. Savoie.
p. cm.
ISBN 978-1-58394-241-3
1. Tae kwon do – Handbooks, manuals, etc. I. Title.
GV1114.9.S28 2009   796.815–dc22   2009053081

1 2 3 4 5 6 7 8 9 Transcontinental – Imprimerie Gagné 14 13 12 11 10

Table of Contents

It is a huge challenge for any author writing about taekwondo to reveal specific know-how with erudition and linguistic skill. Master Gilles R. Savoie is an expert in taekwondo and also a holder of the sixth dan from the Kukkiwon. Most importantly, he is a serious contributor to the taekwondo world.

This book can be recommended to a variety of readers, especially those with an interest in developing their techniques and improving their visualization and nutrition, among others. He is also a reflexologist and has simplified some massage techniques for the convenience of the reader.

Moreover, the sections on the mind, concentration, and mental conditioning provide equally useful knowledge for taekwondo practitioners as well as nonpractitioners. I especially enjoyed the chapter on propulsion versus rotation in hip movements. In this chapter, he proves how impact force is multiplied through a lever action.

This book is an incentive to all taekwondo practitioners to progress in their mental and physical practice. For those with an interest in taekwondo, this book can be considered a stimulus to the world of martial arts.

This book also deserves to be translated in other languages. All kinds of readers can deepen themselves through this material.

Chungwon Choue

– Chungwon Choue

President of the World Taekwondo Federation, 2005

I would like to express appreciation and congratulations to Master Gilles R. Savoie for generously sharing his research, insights, and knowledge to advance taekwondo. By writing Taekwondo: A Technical Manual *he joins the finest martial arts tradition of service through teaching. Master Savoie is clearly committed to the highest taekwondo principles and philosophy. His passion for taekwondo and his commitment to its traditions are the marks of a distinguished and dedicated martial artist and master.*

Using specific principles of physics, Master Savoie demonstrates a hip-propulsion movement that generates great speed, momentum, impetus, and impact. With drawings, graphics, and pictures, the writer offers the reader opportunities to understand, learn, and master this movement. By properly applying the techniques, practitioners can direct their momentum and use technique combinations with great speed and accuracy.

Proper visualization techniques are proven to greatly improve fighting strategies. Master Savoie offers a special visualization technique that can enhance performance by increasing the possibility for practitioners to execute an offensive technique (action) with timing almost as if they had executed a defensive technique or counterattack (reaction).

Respect, sincerity, and discipline are fundamental to Master Savoie's taekwondo teaching style. Through this book, Master Savoie provides you with opportunities for self-discovery as you explore and expand your mental and physical abilities.

Once more, congratulations to Master Gilles R. Savoie for Taekwondo: A Technical Manual.

– Grandmaster Kee Ha, eighth dan
President, Taekwondo Association of Canada

It is with great pleasure and honor that I am writing this foreword for Master Savoie. I am writing not only as a taekwondo student but also as a partner, sharing the same interest in taekwondo movements and their biomechanics.

The human body is a fascinating machine, and studying it is intriguing. One of the things that has always interested me, in my physical education studies as well as in medicine and orthopedics, is biomechanical movement. Enriching discoveries can be made by analyzing and breaking down sequences of body movement. That quest for information can allow us to make some modifications afterward. Generally, we seek to modify a movement in order to improve it and make it more efficient.

Master Gilles R. Savoie definitely has a great passion for biomechanical movement and has completed some very interesting new techniques. The accuracy of his theory on using propulsion instead of the traditional rotation can be confirmed on paper and in practice. His passion and the depth of his knowledge of taekwondo coupled with his work will positively change the practice of the art.

I remember students' reactions when Master Savoie introduced his new technique. Obviously, such drastic changes to a specific movement, which previously had been repeated so often and therefore imprinted on our brains, was not easily accepted. Today, his students, particularly the more advanced, have assimilated these new notions with satisfaction, clearly recognizing their efficiency and relevance.

In addition to explanations and descriptions of his new theories, this book contains a multitude of other facets regarding taekwondo to satisfy the reader. Enjoy the book, and may all of you make great discoveries.

– Dr. Simon Mercier

Student and orthopedic surgeon

The movements used in taekwondo are complex and hard to model. To synchronize all parts of the body to provide both speed and striking power to a particular body part in a short time requires many years of practice and research. Far from limiting himself to the techniques he has learned, Master Gilles R. Savoie has always sought ways to improve them.

You'll find in this book the results of many years of research, carefully condensed and validated with detailed scientific explanations. For the taekwondo practitioner, these detailed techniques will be an indispensable tool for improving performance and optimizing physical and psychological force. For the beginner, this book contains the expertise of a specialist who imparts his passion for martial arts and integrates this expertise into a way of life.

As a physics consultant, it was a great pleasure to discover how passionately science could be put to the service of martial arts to demonstrate the efficiency of certain movements. Like me, by reading this book you will discover a passionate man who was not afraid to submit his theories to the laws of physics and who has come out a winner with the confirmation of his predictions. Congratulations to Master Gilles R. Savoie.

Louis Bujold

– Louis Bujold
Physics teacher

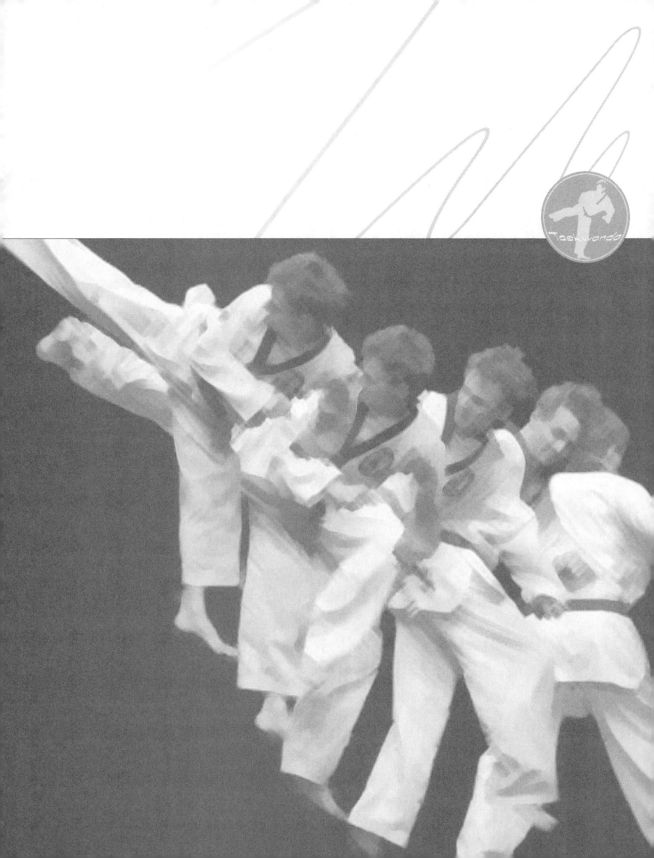

Many people perceive martial arts as violent. In fact, martial arts are for self-defense and sporting combat.

Personally, what attracts me most to martial arts is the practitioners' agility and their outstanding feats in combat. Martial artists demonstrate a power of concentration that greatly impresses me. I began training in martial arts because I wanted to be strong and respected by others. After one year of training, I had obtained my second belt, orange. Thinking that I had learned enough, or rather that there was nothing more to be learned, I stopped going to classes. I continued to practice by myself at home and sparred with other *karatekas* of different styles.

One day, I sparred with a man who had just arrived home after many months of taekwondo training in Korea. He had been exposed to very intense training there, under the direction of well-respected masters. My bout with this practitioner opened my eyes. The way he mastered his energy was spectacular. Every technique performed was precisely timed to attain its objective. At that point I realized that I had not learned the true meaning of martial arts, and I was not feeling the force that governs taekwondo practitioners. This force or energy is the key. After this shocking realization, I returned to my study of martial arts.

How can we channel this energy? How can we increase our level of concentration? I have a strong imagination and have used it since the beginning of my martial arts training. I have always had questions in my mind about the "why" and the "how," and I have searched for answers and explanations within myself. When we are sincere and in contact with our inner soul, it can be very surprising to see the answers to our questions just waiting to emerge.

It is from this constant questioning that I have come to develop the hip-propulsion movement. It is a movement that allows you to place your hips in an unbalanced position that will permit you to toggle both hips while straightening your kicking leg. This toggling movement offers higher speed than conventional hip rotation does. Furthermore, the momentum created by this toggling movement can easily be eliminated, providing better control. From this movement, I have been able to develop a hybrid technique that can, by its quality of reducing the mass projected while executing the technique, increase the speed of execution along with maintaining control.

When we look at two practitioners in competition, we can easily see that in many cases, neither wants to initiate the attack. Often the referee needs to interfere and give warnings to encourage the confrontation. The reason is simple: action time is longer than reaction time. This means that the practitioner who attacks first is disadvantaged by the action time required to perform the technique, compared to the opponent, who will counter using a reaction technique. With a special visualization technique, I can prepare my brain so that my attack technique (action) will be executed in a similar amount of time as a counterattack (reaction).

To attain this I need to optimize my body. Nutrition plays an important part. By observing certain nutritional rules, digestion is facilitated and the body will have considerably fewer toxins to eliminate. Certain combinations of foods help us in our training. Depending on what type of training you are doing, you may need to fuel your nonlactic anaerobic endurance system, lactic anaerobic system, or aerobic system. Following these nutritional combinations will optimize your physical condition. The science of reflexology also becomes an adjunct for improving blood circulation and providing relaxation in order to improve the body's resting time.

To optimize our body systems and to reach balance, we must master our emotions and follow an appropriate training program. We do not have the luxury of separating the physical and the psychological. One of the most challenging fights we will ever have may be with ourselves. Without the unification of the body and mind, we will be defeated.

Taekwondo not only teaches fighting techniques, it also teaches us to discover ourselves as human beings and to attain balance to allow us to live life. Every day, taekwondo offers us a challenge for self-discovery and to find our place in this world. It teaches us how to be real.

Taekwondo: a world to discover.

Enjoy reading this book.

Taekwondo History

For thousands of years, the Korean martial art of taekwondo has been practiced as a martial art, as a sport, and for self-defense. Buddhist principles and combat techniques come together in taekwondo, an art that values fighting abilities as well as mental discipline.

In the beginning, approximately four thousand years ago, people practiced taekwondo as a means to defend themselves against animal attacks. To do so, they developed powerful fighting techniques that could be projected in different directions.

A painting found on a tombstone erected in 37 BC in the Koguryo kingdom, which covered what is now southern Manchuria and the northern Korean Peninsula, clearly depicts two young men engaged in a taekwondo match.

Wanting to entertain his people, the king of the Paekje kingdom, situated along the Han River on the Korean Peninsula from 18 BC to AD 600, organized taekwondo demonstrations. These activities were enjoyed both by soldiers and other citizens.

Taekwondo gained great popularity in the kingdom of Silla, which was in the southeast part of the Korean Peninsula from 57 BC to

AD 936. After having conquered the kingdom of Paekje in 668 and Koguryo in 670, Silla unified the three kingdoms, which Silla and its successors maintained for three hundred years. King Jinheung was responsible for unifying the three kingdoms and organizing a military group, the Hwa Rang Do. Military, educational, and social values were taught to the young noblemen who made up the Hwa Rang Do, and they devoted themselves to the development of their minds and bodies to better serve their kingdom. Their martial spirit was a source of inspiration for the whole nation. They followed a code of honor that included loyalty to the nation, respect and obedience to their parents, courage during combat, and wisdom when using force or, when necessary, taking life. This code of honor is present in a different form today: in taekwondo training.

The study of unarmed combat increased in popularity during the Koryo dynasty (935 to 1392). In this period the martial art was called *Soo Bak Do*, and it was practiced as a sport with detailed rules as well as a form of martial art with a military purpose. The masters of Soo Bak Do used scientific principles to improve the fighting techniques of the art. Soo Bak Do's popularity allowed the royal family to support and encourage its practice, and often those who distinguished themselves in the art were favored or promoted in both civil and military matters. The Koryo king organized Soo Bak Do events and demonstrations each year.

At the end of the Koryo dynasty, Buddhism was no longer the state religion; King Taejo, founder of the Yi dynasty in 1392, chose Confucianism instead, and consequently the importance of military training, physical conditioning, and the ability to defend the nation was diminished. With the adoption of Confucian ideas, new importance was placed on learning classical Chinese culture, while physical activities were underappreciated. The result was that men of higher social classes now passed the time by reading Chinese classical texts, composing poetry, and practicing music; physical activities were only practiced by lower-class men. Taekwondo, known in those days by the name *Tae Kyon*, was losing popularity. Military officers received no recognition at the social or political level. The situation was the exact opposite of what it had been in the previous dynasty.

A change was soon to come with the arrival of King Chongjo, who showed interest in martial arts. In 1790 he ordered General Lee Duck Mu to compile a manual on all martial arts that existed in Korea. This manual rapidly became a classic. Even with his involvement, King Chongjo did not succeed in reversing the disinterest that his people showed for martial arts. But thanks to his manual, the techniques of the martial arts were preserved for future generations.

With this disinterest in martial arts and an emphasis instead on military activities, neglect of national defense continued during the eighteenth and nineteenth centuries. There were no organized martial arts schools, and techniques were taught by father to son or by instructors to disciples in secret. The weakness of the military made the country vulnerable. In 1909, Japan invaded Korea and took control. During the occupation, martial arts were forbidden. Having no arms to defend themselves, some Koreans continued to practice Tae Kyon in secret, and in this way Tae Kyon continued to survive and became even stronger. It was an important tool for Koreans to maintain their identity, values, and courage.

Along with the invasion, Koreans came into contact with a Japanese martial art, karate, as well as other Chinese martial arts. Many of their techniques were incorporated into Tae Kyon by Koreans, creating different styles of the art built on the principles of the Tang Soo Do and Kong Soo Do martial arts.

After the liberation of Korea in 1945, Koreans were again able to practice their martial arts openly. The Japanese occupation had considerably modified the Korean martial arts, and so many masters were reunited to combine the different styles developed during the occupation; this was an effort to recover traditional Tae Kyon as it had been prior to the influence of Japanese karate or Chinese styles on Korean culture. After many years of meetings and debates, the directors of the six most influential Korean schools came to an agreement on standardizing the technical teaching methods. *Taekwondo* was the name chosen to represent this new martial art. In Korean, *tae* means strikes delivered with the feet, *kwon* means strikes delivered with the fists, and *do* means the martial philosophy, the way of life.

As the country was now free, taekwondo could develop at the level of a sport. In October 1962 it was made an official activity at the Forty-third Korean National Games. In 1964 Master Chong Lee came to Canada to teach this martial art. He opened various schools

In Korean, *tae* means strikes delivered with the feet, *kwon* means strikes delivered with the fists, and *do* means the martial philosophy, the way of life.

in Quebec that extended into neighboring provinces and nurtured many world champions. Master Gilles R. Savoie became his student and later developed this martial art on the Gaspé Peninsula in the eastern part of Quebec.

In January 1971 Dr. Un Young Kim was elected president of the Korean Taekwondo Association. He was deeply involved in the development of the discipline and wanted to raise awareness of taekwondo and make it the Korean national sport. In May 1973 he organized the World Taekwondo Federation to structure the evolution of the art to an international level. Under his presidency, the Kukkiwon was built in Seoul. The name means "national sports institute," and the Kukkiwon became the world taekwondo training headquarters. In 1975 the World Taekwondo Federation became official at the General Assembly of International Sports Federations. Taekwondo became an official sport at the International Military Sports Council in 1976. And in 1980 taekwondo was elevated to an Olympic sport by the International Olympic Committee. On June 11, 2004, Dr. Chungwon Choue was nominated president of the World Taekwondo Federation. He created a reform committee with the goal of making the sport more exciting and appealing to global audiences by revamping the sport's world governing body.

Taekwondo enjoys wide popularity mainly due to the visibly spectacular feats in sparring, board-breaking demonstrations, and self-defense. We also now know that Buddhist techniques of meditation and concentration elevated taekwondo to a superior level from that of a simple sport.

Taekwondo is an official discipline in the Pan-American Games and in the Olympic Games. Its spiritual side, its relationship with meditation techniques, and its nonviolent Buddhist principles intrigue and attract more and more enthusiasts. In the modern world, where stress takes an increasing toll on us and with self-realization hard to attain, traditional taekwondo has the potential to extend its history for the well-being of its enthusiasts.

Taekwondo Ethics

MODESTY

SELF-CONTROL

PERSEVERANCE

SOME PRINCIPLES TO REMEMBER

- Discipline

- Respect

- Sincerity

- Never encourage violence

- Respect nature

- Train the spirit and the body

- Promote friendly relations

- Be a courageous opponent of what is false

TAEKWONDO TERMS AND DEFINITIONS

TAE	foot strike
KWON	fist strike
DO	life philosophy

From these definitions, we can establish fundamental taekwondo concepts. We know that in practicing this art we use techniques employing the feet and hands. A student can easily come to think that he or she has mastered these fundamental movements in a few months of training, but it is impossible to learn how to execute them with force, timing, and efficiency in such a short time.

The taekwondo ethic of **self-control** should be among the main goals of practicing the art because one of the biggest obstacles we may encounter will be how to master ourselves. Every challenge that we overcome will bring us one step closer to this mastery, elevating us to a higher level of energy. I am talking about mastering ourselves on the physical level as well as on the mental level. Knowing that an excellent way to train the spirit is to train the physical body, the student must practice regularly and concentrate as much as possible on the details of the execution of every single technique.

The student needs to use visualization techniques to feel the energy travel through the body down to the extremities that are executing the technique. In the "Visualization" chapter you will see why I've placed **modesty** among the taekwondo ethics; this quality elevates visualization techniques to a special level.

Taking these elements into consideration, the student must execute the techniques repeatedly, analyzing him – or herself and adding details in the visualization field to allow the sensation of the technique to become more than simply emotional. Even if the results seem slow to appear, the student must persevere and remember that the attitude developed by including all the details in the execution of the technique is as important as the technique itself. This is why I've included **perseverance** among the taekwondo ethics. The student's mind will associate this attitude with the execution of the technique, which will greatly influence its force. We know that what gives life to a technique is the energy that animates it.

The force developed is the result of the way in which we have allowed the union of the technique and its energy. We must therefore take a stance that allows us to transfer our center of gravity in a way that we execute the technique as we exhale. All the parts of the body must be in harmony to permit the synchronization of muscular contractions required to transfer energy from their source to the technique without creating pointless resistance, which would have an effect similar to an electrical short circuit.

The taekwondo practitioner needs to assume a combat position that allows him or her, at certain times, to execute techniques while supporting the weight of the body on only one foot, and at other times to position the body in a way that allows a transition in which there is no contact with the floor to deliver an attack or a counterattack. The mastery of this balance becomes a very important asset. To achieve it, depending on the circumstances, the center of gravity could be high, low, or more on one foot than the other. For certain techniques, it is even necessary to shift the center of gravity outside our two-footed stance.

We are able to walk because we constantly transfer our center of gravity forward. As soon as the center of gravity stops moving, we stop walking. A person walks fluidly because the center of gravity is transferred at a constant speed; otherwise our gait would be stilted like a primitive robot's. This mastery of the stability of our center of gravity allows us to move. So in reality, what allows us to walk is that we constantly shift our center of gravity. We put ourselves in an unbalanced position, and then try to gain balance; as soon as we succeed, we put ourselves in an unbalanced position again. To achieve movement, there must be an imbalance. In order to grow mentally, we must equally experience a certain amount of imbalance. The orbits of the planets and the movement of the heavens exist in part because there is an unbalanced force; otherwise there would be nothing. It is by seeking to attain balance that a cycle develops to allow the universe to evolve, as it is for human beings.

Combat in taekwondo must be seen as a kind of dance. Our opponent should be considered more as our dance partner. We must dance with our opponent, and there must be an energy that develops, allowing a certain dynamic to take form so that the action of one will provoke the reaction of the other, and vice versa. A constant reevaluation of the situation must take place to permit an attack or a reorientation for counterattack. To attain that stage, sparring moves to heightened concentration, which elevates the practitioner to a level of consciousness that allows him or her to feel the opponent's displacement. It becomes possible to execute techniques with a fluidity of movement and a high degree of precision while expending minimal energy. A well-trained student will know when to attack the opponent by studying the changes in his or her center of gravity.

Basic Principles

FORCE AND SPEED

Excellent muscle strength is imperative to provide protection for the vital organs against impact.

One important factor is speed:
striking force = mass × speed, or *F = MV*.

Let's compare muscle mass to a four-inch ball weighing two pounds. Clearly two pounds is not a large mass. Place a four-inch-square piece of glass horizontally on four small cubes, one at each corner to support the glass. Position the two-pound ball on the glass, and the glass will easily support the ball's weight without breaking. If the same two-pound ball falls onto the glass from three feet above it, however, the glass will break.

This demonstrates that mass without speed (velocity) represents less force than if it acquires speed. Speed has a multiplying factor that increases striking force. This principle is of the utmost importance in understanding taekwondo techniques. The formula **striking force = mass × speed** is very basic: double the speed and the striking force increases. To achieve this result, the technique must also be precise. This concept will be covered in more depth in the "Hip Movement" chapter.

> **Note : In this book, I have used the formula F=MV.**
>
> In order to facilitate understanding of the movement, **F** represents the striking force, **M** is the concentrated mass at the point of impact, and **V** is the speed at which the mass is displaced (see the "Formulas" chapter).

CONCENTRATING STRIKING FORCE

With your right thumb, try to push with a certain amount of force into the palm of your left hand. Pay particular attention to the pain you feel in your left palm.

Now imagine that you have a needle with a sharp point touching the palm of your left hand. Think about pushing the needle against your palm with the same force that you used with your thumb. It is easy to imagine the pain this would cause.

In both examples, the same force is applied from the right thumb. When concentrated in a smaller area, the pain is not the same. Concentrated force will cause more damage. It is imperative to know the importance of concentrating our striking force in a small area. But where do we get the force required ?

Your largest energy reservoir, located in the abdomen, becomes an important ally. From the movement described in the "Hip Movement" chapter, you have the potential to concentrate the energy from that reservoir into a single point and to make it travel with a wave effect to the target extremity of the technique. Shifting your center of gravity to maintain a controlled unbalanced position is imperative. I say "controlled" because balance must be attained at the moment the technique has reached its final execution point.

Having contributed to the concentration of force into a precise point at a precise time, the muscles must be relaxed instantly, and the body must again be placed into an unbalanced position to prepare for the next action.

THE ROLE OF MUSCLE POWER

Excellent muscle tone along with muscular equilibrium are essential for executing movements without getting injured. We must develop muscle resistance in both strength and flexibility. The training objective is to develop muscles capable of contracting and relaxing quickly.

We saw previously that the faster the technique, the greater the striking force. The same formula, **striking force = mass × speed**, applies to muscle contractions. Therefore, the faster the muscles contract, the greater the striking force that is developed. This is physics.

STRIKING FORCE = muscle mass × speed of the technique

In this example, I've modified the formula to simplify understanding the importance of muscle contraction speed:

STRIKING MUSCLE FORCE (muscle power) = muscle mass × speed of muscle contraction

Consequently, our striking force can be increased on two levels:

FIRST, the technique must be executed as quickly as possible, and to do so it must travel the shortest distance toward the target – in a straight line.

SECOND, the muscle force must be perfectly developed to produce rapid contraction.

MUSCLE ENERGY

Energy is needed for muscle contraction. That energy must be in the form of adenosine triphosphate (ATP). The human body has three systems that produce ATP:

• ALACTIC ANAEROBIC SYSTEM

This system supplies very intense strength. It permits rapid movement because muscle cells already have a small amount of ATP. When that reserve is consumed, creatine phosphate, also present in small quantities in muscle cells, releases its energy to produce ATP. This allows a series of maximum muscular contractions for an average of ten seconds. The advantage of this system is that it does not produce lactic acid even in the absence of oxygen, which is why it can produce ATP during maximum muscular contraction.

• LACTIC ACID ANAEROBIC SYSTEM

Glycogen in the muscles becomes the only source for producing ATP in a strong muscular contraction. This system cannot operate for more than twenty seconds without producing lactic acid. If a high-intensity effort exceeds 120 seconds, the muscles will no longer be able to perform due to the high accumulation of lactic acid.

• AEROBIC SYSTEM

The aerobic system can produce ATP in large amounts for a relatively long time. In order to do so, muscular contraction must be relatively weak. The advantage is that it does not cause lactic acid to accumulate in muscle cells.

In some sports, developing a single system may be acceptable, but in taekwondo we need to have strength in all three systems. Before beginning training, we must have a strong aerobic foundation. Later, the other two systems may be developed through specific exercises. Once aerobic endurance has been achieved through continual training, the student can train in intervals. With a strong aerobic endurance system, the recuperation time in interval training will be shorter.

I won't go into detail about these training systems, since there are excellent books that cover them. What I want to point out are the distinct exercise programs for each of the systems that produce ATP. It is important to put the required effort into developing each system. The overall body system requires a strong foundation in aerobic endurance.

RHYTHM

An essential element in executing the techniques of taekwondo is rhythm. The execution of every technique has specific timing. The planet earth takes 365.25 days to make one orbit around the sun. The moon takes 27.32 days to orbit the earth. The earth makes one rotation on its axis in 23 hours and 56 minutes. This information provides the idea of a cycle. Lost rhythm means wasted energy, but maintaining rhythm does not mean jumping around like a kangaroo. I am referring to being conscious of the rhythm of our breathing, the shifts in our center of gravity, and so on. All of these together allow us to execute our movements with greater speed.

In addition, we must be conscious of our opponent's rhythm, which will allow us to anticipate his or her movements and to orient the shift of our center of gravity to respond quickly and adequately. This rhythm allows muscle relaxation to prepare for rapid contraction.

Pumsae, choreography in which the student executes sparring techniques facing an imaginary opponent using precise timing and orientation, becomes an exercise in which concentration, breathing, balance, and rhythm are practiced. In Pumsae, rhythm allows combinations of movements without stopping the mind. It could be compared to dancing the tango. At first, the student must concentrate on each movement to master it. With time, as the student's abilities and rhythm are developed, a fluidity in movement allows movement with minimum energy. After being executed repeatedly, these movements will develop the person intellectually, elevating the mind to another level. The movements become more precise and gracious. In addition, executing Pumsae increases the taekwondo practitioner's power of concentration. Pumsae is thus an excellent exercise to practice:

- **self-defense techniques**

- **power of concentration**

- **rhythm**

- **synchronization**

The practice of synchronizing all these elements in the execution of Pumsae teaches the student to bring the concentration level to a point where the mind will be able to concentrate on all the tasks required to execute them in an ordered fashion without allowing distraction by useless information.

SYNCHRONIZATION

Synchronization is similar to conducting an orchestra. If there is a rhythm for every technique executed, then surely there is synchronization. Imagine listening to a thirty-piece orchestra. Each performer may have excellent rhythm, but if there is no synchronization, there will be no melody. In taekwondo, if there is no synchronization, the released energy that originates from the abdomen will not reach the technique's extremity. This can be compared to a golfer whose stroke has no synchronization; the ball will not travel far.

For the student of taekwondo, a technique without synchronization will produce a muffled low-frequency sound when the striking-glove target is hit, similar to the energy used to push a heavy object. With good synchronization, the sound will be high-pitched and faster, similar to the sound produced by a whip strike.

When a movement without synchronization is used in sparring, the opponent can easily absorb the energy delivered by the technique and convert it into motion, eliminating potential pain from the strike. When a synchronized technique is delivered, the opponent will have more difficulty absorbing the energy to transform it into movement because of its high speed. Consequently, he will feel the energy deeply in the form of pain.

Hip Movement: Hip Rotation or Hip Propulsion?

The study of taekwondo reflects the laws of physics. What students are searching for is often a way to develop the maximum striking force of every technique using the least possible energy.

I have studied martial arts for forty years, earning black belts in karate, jujitsu, and taekwondo. I have observed the performance of many black belts along with the teaching of many instructors. In a general way, students are taught to use a hip-rotation movement to execute a technique with force. This movement develops a good striking force.

To obtain my sixth dan in taekwondo, I wrote a paper describing a hip movement that I have developed. This movement is a hip propulsion that allows us to bring the hip to a point where another hip movement – this time a toggle movement – can be added to the technique, developing an increase in speed with an increase in striking force and control. This movement then permits many technique combinations that are difficult and perhaps impossible to execute with a hip-rotation movement.

For now, let's study a popular basic technique in taekwondo: *Bichagi*. Many people call this a circular kick. We often hear

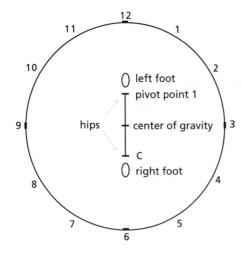

Figure 1 : The clock

Figure 2 : Hip rotation

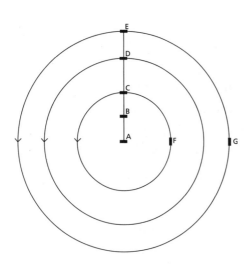

instructors tell students, "Turn your hips." Instructors repeatedly tell students to turn their hips if they want to develop force, and often students ask instructors, "Why will turning my hips help me develop force?" You would be surprised to hear the variety of answers that I've heard instructors give that show a lack of knowledge of the laws of physics.

I will share a teaching method that I've developed to help my students understand the reasons and the need for the hip movements necessary to execute taekwondo techniques. To simplify the explanations in the following paragraphs, I'll refer to the *Bichagi*, executed with the right leg, standing on the floor with the left foot forward.

In all of my classes, I have changed the term *turn* in the case of turning the hip to *propel*. To explain the orientation of the hip, I use the numbers of the clock face. Twelve o'clock represents the highest point of the hip as seen from a position looking from above toward the floor and pointing toward the target.

In the combat position shown in **Figure 1**, the practitioner is standing with the left foot pointed toward 12 o'clock to execute a *Bichagi*. From pivot point 1, you must move your hip, at point C and pointing toward 6 o'clock, to the 1 o'clock position, turning counterclockwise. The manner in which you move your hip to the position corresponding to 1 o'clock is extremely important. You must not think about turning your hip; you must instead move it to the 1 o'clock position as quickly as possible, moving in a straight line with a movement I call **propulsion**.

At this point, your knee is bent, and your toes point toward the floor. Your knee will unbend, executing the *Bichagi*. During this movement, your hip will toggle from the 1 o'clock position to the 12 o'clock position. The toggling movement is aided by the supporting left leg. Once the 12 o'clock position is reached, the technique has reached its final point, and the technique is complete.

Here, the critical point is from 1 o'clock to 12 o'clock. Your hip must bring your knee to the 1 o'clock position to permit the leg to straighten while it moves to the 12 o'clock position. This is the fundamental way the *Bichagi* should be executed. Why? Here is where physics makes the technique interesting. Let's take a closer look at **hip rotation** in **Figure 2**.

Consider a combat position where your left leg is in front. This means that your right hip, at point A, is supported by your left leg resting on the floor. With the support of your left leg, your hip at point C can make a 360-degree rotation from point A, drawing a circle on the floor. Your right leg is aligned with point C, drawing a larger circle on the floor. The hip rotation draws circle F from point C on the floor while your foot draws circle G from point E.

For now, let's say that in Figure 2 the distance between point A and point C, which represents the width of the hip, is 4 inches. This means that circle F has a radius of 4 inches. To simplify, let's say that in this example, your leg has a length of 39 inches. This length added to the radius of circle F gives 43 inches for the radius of circle G. Using the equation **C = 2πr**, where **C** is the circumference, **π** is the constant 3.14, and **r** is the radius, we can calculate the circumference of circle F as 2 × 3.14 × 4 = 25 inches. From this same equation, the circumference of circle G is 2 × 3.14 × 43 = 270 inches. Knowing both circumferences, we can compare that of circle F with that of circle G, which is 11 times longer.

Let's return to Figure 1. Imagine being in the position where you have just finished executing a *Bichagi*: you are standing on your left leg with your right leg completely stretched, the right hip corner pointing toward 12 o'clock and aligned with your leg and foot. Apply this position to Figure 2. This means that point A in Figure 2 represents your left supporting leg, and point E represents your right foot, pointing at 12 o'clock. In this case, let's assume the force applied at point C in Figure 2 is 110 newtons. What will be the force applied or delivered at point E? Since there is no lever action and the right leg is directly attached to the right hip, the force at point E is exactly the same as at point C.

We know that energy cannot be created nor destroyed. But it is important to understand that energy can be transformed. If we want to drive a nail into a piece of wood, we must use the weight of a hammer. The weight of the hammer on its own is not sufficient to drive the nail into the piece of wood; we must add a movement that will give speed to the hammer's weight or mass. All of these forces, once well synchronized, will generate the required energy to drive the nail into the piece of wood.

Let's look again at the *Bichagi* technique once the right leg is completely stretched out. Like the hammer in the previous example, this leg represents a mass at point E in Figure 2. We now know that a mass must undergo movement in order to generate more force. Consider, for example, that it takes 1 second to complete circle F in Figure 2 from a hip rotation at point A. Since the circumference of circle G is 11 times longer than that of circle F, how many seconds will it take to complete circle G? At first glance it may seem surprising, but the time required is exactly the same as that required to complete circle F. These circles are all made with the same hip rotation, so no matter how much more length is added to the radius from point C in Figure 2, the time required to complete the hip rotation will be exactly the same as the time required to draw the circle at point C. The difference between circle F and circle G in Figure 2 is that circle G has 11 times more distance to cover than circle F. To accomplish this, the speed must be 11 times faster. The point of these examples is **speed**.

A greater force is generated when movement, or speed, is applied. The equation **striking force = mass × speed** clearly explains this concept. It is clear that the foot at point E in Figure 2 travels rapidly. The force generated will be greater, but it will have the same mass.

At this point the question that should interest any student is, how can we achieve maximum speed? Previously, I said that I had changed the term *rotate* to *propel*. You'll understand why in the following discussion.

In order to walk, you must put yourself in an unbalanced position by shifting your center of gravity in the direction you want to go. You can walk if you continually shift your center of gravity forward. As

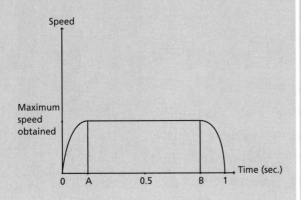

Figure 3 : Speed over time

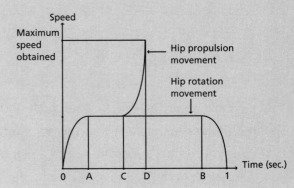

Figure 4 : Speed over time with hip rotation

soon as balance is established, you stop walking. The same principle applies for the *Bichagi*. If you want speed, meaning if you want point C in Figure 2 to travel as fast as possible on circle F, your hip must be placed in an unbalanced position. When the hip seeks its balanced position, your body will be arranged to move at very high speed.

To produce this speed, the right hip in Figure 1 must point toward 1 o'clock. When the hip is propelled as far forward as possible, pointing toward 1 o'clock, it is ready to toggle. This is aided by the supporting left leg, reaching its point of balance and locked in a position pointing toward 12 o'clock. Here, your principal preoccupation should be from a left combat position, as in Figure 1, to move the right hip from the point facing 6 o'clock toward the point facing 1 o'clock. Then, with the help of the left supporting leg, the right hip will toggle to lock itself pointing toward 12 o'clock. You can see that this movement is not a hip rotation.

Now focus your attention on a hip movement: execute a rotation movement at point C in Figure 2 from the supported point A, with the intention of delivering a *Bichagi* in which the right hip in Figure 1 will start at the 6 o'clock position and stop at 12 o'clock.

In **Figure 3**, I have drawn a curve representing the **speed at which the hip travels over time**, assuming that the complete rotation

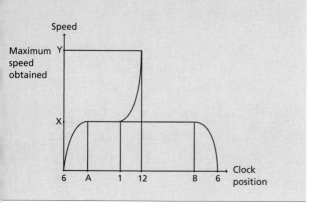

You will need to use figures 1-5 again later in the book. You might want to copy them on a piece of paper so that you can easily refer to them as you read.

Figure 5 : Speed by clock position

is accomplished in 1 second. Remember that in order to produce movement, the center of gravity, point B in Figure 2, must seek balance without attaining it. Notice that speed is maintained for a relatively long period of time. This means that the *Bichagi* can be executed between point A and point B in Figure 3. In this example, we are still talking about a hip-rotation movement, in which the right hip in Figure 1 can never be pushed forward to its unbalanced point to face 1 o'clock. Consequently, the hip will not find its balanced point – since it never lost it – and aided by the left supporting leg will lock itself at a point facing 12 o'clock, which, as discussed previously, is the point where the hip can travel at its greatest speed.

Let's draw a curve over Figure 3 to represent the propelled hip movement, which we can observe in **Figure 4**. Here we see that a greater speed develops, but the problem is in the fact that the speed on the y-axis is attained in a very short period of time, forcing the practitioner to be extremely precise in executing the technique. In Figure 4 it must start at time C and must be completed at time D. You'll understand why in the following discussion.

Let's draw the same curve representing speed, but instead of speed over time, we will use the clock principle from Figure 1. In **Figure 5** the curve is **speed by clock position**, where the numbers correspond to the clock positions in Figure 1. In Figure 5, we see that great speed can be developed from a rotation movement, a curve from 6 o'clock to 6 o'clock, but much greater speed can be achieved from a propelled movement, a curve from 1 o'clock to 12 o'clock.

The hip rotation and propulsion movements look relatively similar. To bring the right hip, point C in Figure 1, from the 6 o'clock position to its forward point at 1 o'clock, we should not think of a hip-rotation movement but rather of a propulsion movement. We can clearly see that the critical time is when the right hip in Figure 1 is between the 1 o'clock and 12 o'clock positions. This signifies that up to the 1 o'clock position, the hip must propel the leg, knee bent, toes pointing to the floor. You must only begin to straighten your leg when the right hip moves from its unbalanced position facing 1 o'clock to its balanced position, locking itself to face 12 o'clock, at which position the technique is complete.

To develop high speed, energy must travel like a wave from hip point C in Figure 2 up to foot point E. In this case, the speed of the knee at point D is multiplied by the radius from point C to point D. The speed at point D is multiplied by the radius from point D to point E. For example, what is the force represented at point E in Figure 2 when the 12 o'clock position is reached? The striking force at point C is **striking force = mass × speed,** where mass represents the hip mass. Therefore, at point C, we have the mass of the hip multiplied by the speed, which gives the striking force at point C. At point D, we have **striking force D = mass × speed,** where the mass at point D is multiplied by the speed developed by the muscular energy required to move point D to the 1 o'clock position. At point E, we have **striking force E = mass × speed,** where the mass is multiplied by the speed developed by the muscular energy necessary to straighten the leg. At this point, muscular energy is very significant, since it is developed by the quadriceps. Take a closer look at the equation **striking force = mass × speed.** Notice that when mass and speed are at their greatest, the force developed is greater. In Figure 2, the greatest speed is attained at point E, partly because point E travels at a different speed than point D, which in turn travels at a different speed than point C. If the energy travels in the correct way, using the various pivot points to increase the radius to in turn increase speed, the striking force is extremely powerful and can be focused at a very precise point at a precise time. *This implies a hip-propulsion movement.*

In this section, I applied the hip-propulsion movement using the *Bichagi* technique to simplify understanding of this special movement. The same principle can be applied to the majority of taekwondo techniques. The difference will be in the orientation of the hip position as it relates to the clock positions. You need to propel your hip where it will be at the point to toggle from an unbalanced point to a balanced point, locking itself in the required position according to the clock position. The kicking technique then must be executed during the toggle, as explained with the *Bichagi* technique. The details of each technique are described in the "Fundamental Techniques" chapter.

COMBINATIONS

By this point you will probably agree that if you execute a kicking technique using the hip-rotation movement, you develop less striking force than if you had mastered and used the hip-propulsion movement. Some practitioners may not believe that an increase in striking force is required, since the striking force developed in the hip-rotation movement is powerful enough in most situations, and succeeds in most cases to considerably destabilize the opponent. Incompetition, the objective is not necessarily to cause injury to your opponent, as opposed to a street self-defense situation in which your life could be in danger. In competition, however, we must score, and to do so we must reach the target as often as possible.

Based on the information provided in the previous section, it should be obvious that the time required to execute a foot technique from beginning to end is not that much faster when delivered by a hip-propulsion movement compared to a hip-rotation movement. But since the propulsion movement's mass is transferred only at the end – that is to say, at the beginning of the toggling movement where the speed is the greatest – the striking force developed by this propulsion movement is much greater than that delivered by the hip-rotation movement. At this point the only advantage to the propulsion movement over the rotation movement appears to be the striking force, not the speed of execution. However, there are further advantages besides what we have covered so far.

INERTIA, MOMENTUM, AND IMPETUS

Definitions:

- **Inertia is the body's resistance, relative to its mass, to oppose movement.**

- **Momentum is mass in movement.**

- **Impetus is change of momentum.**

When you're driving and you have to stop quickly by applying the brakes, the force that pushes your body forward is created by impetus. In taekwondo, if you execute the *Bichagi* technique from a hip-rotation movement, your leg will acquire momentum, and if your opponent moves slightly to avoid your attack, this momentum will place you in an unbalanced position. This imbalance creates vulnerability and offers your opponent the opportunity to attack you. Since every action provokes a reaction, and the momentum developed while executing the *Bichagi* technique forces you to continue your movement in the same direction, you need to take this into consideration when you want to execute a combination of techniques.

For example, say you want to execute a combination of techniques. After having started your *Bichagi* technique, you realize that a *Dwi Chagi* would work well as a combination technique following the *Bichagi*, since the *Dwi Chagi* can easily use the inertia developed by the *Bichagi* to its advantage. The weakness of this technique is that an experienced opponent will suspect such an obvious combination, and he or she then has the opportunity to prepare to receive the *Dwi Chagi* once the *Bichagi* has been thrown. For your opponent, this is as simple as 2 + 2 = 4. Techniques from a hip-rotation movement used in combination are easily predictable.

With the hip-propulsion movement followed by the toggling movement, the momentum you develop is easy to readjust. To understand why, look at Figure 5 again. Remember that the hip was placed in imbalance at the point corresponding to 1 o'clock. This was when the hip sought its balance, which is between the 1 o'clock and 12 o'clock positions while the leg was straightened to execute the *Bichagi*. We must remember that what allowed the hip to toggle was the assistance of the left leg supported by the floor. In this way, it is easy to relax the left hip to allow the right hip in Figure 1, facing the 12 o'clock position in Figure 5, to retract slightly. This slight retraction is largely sufficient to neutralize the effect of momentum. Once momentum is neutralized, you have a multitude of possibilities. You can rapidly return your kicking leg to its original position to prevent any counterattack from your opponent. If you want to execute a technique combination after delivering a *Bichagi*, you now have several more choices in addition to the *Dwi Chagi*, since you can bring your leg back to its original position at very high speed and continue with another technique while turning backward. In other words, you can attack clockwise with an initial technique and combine it with a second counterclockwise technique. Even for an experienced opponent, such a combination can be very difficult, if not impossible, to anticipate.

Once the right hip in Figure 1 has retracted after having completed the *Bichagi* technique, it is now facing the 1 o'clock position. This is the start of the toggling movement in which great speed is developed in the *Bichagi* technique. The hip is therefore well placed to start over again, to deliver another *Bichagi* at high speed, or to deliver some other technique; a huge choice of techniques becomes available. If you decide not to use a second technique while using the hip-propulsion movement, you can simply use the speed that you developed while seeking balance by putting your leg on the floor after having slightly retracted your hip to reposition yourself, which allows your displacement to prevent a counterattack from your opponent.

For example, you are in a combat position with your left leg forward while your opponent is in a combat position also with the left leg forward. Your opponent attacks with a *Bichagi* but suspects that you are waiting for the attack and ready to make a counterattack. If you haven't mastered the hip-propulsion movement, you risk hesitancy in performing your technique. If you do it with a hip-rotation movement, more power is applied and more momentum develops. Consequently, your imbalance will be greater if your opponent avoids it and then counters. With all this momentum, a counterattack from your opponent will be disastrous because it is now practically impossible for you to correct your imbalance to transform the force of impact into movement. This leaves the only choice to absorb the blast, causing injury or at the very least great pain. In contrast, if you master the hip-propulsion movement, you know you can neutralize the effect of the momentum.

In the above example, you can execute a powerful *Bichagi* without hesitation. As soon as the technique is completed, once the effect of the momentum is neutralized, you can then place your leg on the floor with most of your center of gravity on it to allow your final position to be 90 degrees to your opponent. From this position, a second strong offensive becomes possible, even if your opponent tries to counter.

The hip-propulsion movement communicates movement only to the smaller mass of the kicking leg, contrary to a rotation movement, which puts the larger mass of the whole body into action. The hip-propulsion movement permits greater speed to be created rapidly in the kicking foot in a short period of time. This gives you the ability to modify your strategy and to increase its efficiency. The movement also offers many displacement possibilities after the execution of a technique.

Hybrid Technique

Once you master the hip-propulsion movement, many other possibilities become available. Remember our physics formula: *striking force = mass × speed.* The element that cannot be neglected is speed. When sparring with an opponent it would be disastrous to decrease the speed of our execution. Similarly, if an airplane loses too much speed, it crashes. In taekwondo it is impossible to consider decreasing the speed of execution, as it is too valuable. Speed is the main component of this martial art.

Let's transform the equation as follows: **speed = striking force ÷ mass.** Shown in this way, it is clear that the greater the mass, the lower the speed. This means that if the mass is decreased by half, the speed doubles. Things are getting interesting, wouldn't you agree? We certainly don't want to reduce the mass significantly, because even if we gain in speed, we will lose striking force. We only need to reduce the mass slightly to have a considerable effect on speed. What is lost in force is negligible; you'll understand why in the following explanation.

As discussed above, the striking force developed from a hip-rotation movement is considerable, but the striking force developed from a hip-propulsion movement is much greater. In hip propulsion, we can allow ourselves to decrease the force slightly if this allows us to develop a greater advantage in speed. The obvious problem is that we must reduce the mass. To achieve this, it is out of the question to decrease our muscle mass, which is too important in executing techniques. Nor can we reduce the radius of our technique, because it depends on the length. Obviously we cannot decrease the length of our extremities by cutting off part of a leg. So what can we do to reduce the mass?

Before I answer that, I want to advise you that you must first master the hip-propulsion movement described above before trying to execute the hybrid technique I'm about to explain.

Previously, I explained that for your hip to toggle, you must propel it forward, and in the example of the *Bichagi* technique executed with the right leg, the hip must face the 1 o'clock position to be able to toggle to the 12 o'clock position. Two questions:

1. **Can you propel the hip to the 12 o'clock position before toggling it to the 11 o'clock position?**

2. **Can you propel the hip to the 2 o'clock position before toggling it to the 12 o'clock position?**

If you find the answers, you have understood the principle of the hip-propulsion movement. To answer the first question, you cannot propel your hip toward the 12 o'clock position without a toggle of the lower hip, point A in Figure 2, from the supporting leg. Likewise, if you toggle the hip at point A, it will not be possible to toggle it again, and what remains possible in the technique will be developed from a hip-rotation movement. Try it: from a combat position with your left leg forward, slowly propel your right hip as far forward as you can without toggling the left hip at point A in Figure 2. Looking down at your pelvis, imagine a clock drawn on the floor. By extending an imaginary line across your pelvis through both hips, you should see that the imaginary line extending from your right hip at point C in Figure 2 points to 1 o'clock, if 12 o'clock represents the target or opponent.

To answer the second question, place yourself again into a combat position with your left leg forward, and place yourself in the center of the clock drawn on the floor so that 12 o'clock still points toward your opponent or target. Slowly propel your right hip in Figure 1 to the 1 o'clock position. By toggling both hips at the same time, the farthest distance the right hip can travel is to reach the 12 o'clock position. I explained previously that the distance traveled by the toggling hip is very short, which partially explains the great speed that is developed. The distance usually never exceeds the distance from one hour to the next on the clock in Figure 1. If you push your hip to cover a longer distance than one hour, your hip at point A will no longer be able to toggle from your supporting leg, necessitating a hip-rotation movement of the upper hip at point C in Figure 2.

If you repeat this exercise slowly, you should notice that the hip, once toggled, has the tendency to lock itself, and this happens after it has reached the 12 o'clock position. The hip's physiology is responsible for this effect. You'll notice that there's a slight forward displacement of the hip as it toggles. Place your right hip in Figure 1 facing the 2 o'clock position. Next, displace your right hip from 2 o'clock to the 12 o'clock position. You should notice a big difference from the previous exercise. It is obvious that in order to travel such a distance, greater than one hour on the clock, the right hip in Figure 1 needs to execute a rotation movement, and so no toggling occurs and no slight forward displacement is visible.

This answers the second question. It is impossible to use a toggling movement to displace the upper hip a distance greater than one clock hour, since it is important to properly align with the target. To move a distance greater than one hour, the supporting leg starts to be used as a reference, and so the right hip rotates on the supporting leg.

Based on this information, is it possible to propel the right hip to the 2 o'clock position and toggle the hips to bring the right hip to 1 o'clock? I'd be happy if you'd thought of this question. If you didn't, consider it. One possible answer is that if your opponent is in line with 12 o'clock, and since the technique should be complete once it has reached the 1 o'clock position, the opponent cannot be reached. Additionally, if you execute a *Bichagi* from the 2 o'clock position to 1 o'clock, the main striking vector is more vertical than horizontal. But these two answers, while interesting, bring up problems that can be corrected, which I will explain later. First, I want to give you the correct answer.

TOGGLING THE HIP

This technique must be delivered while the hip is toggling to develop maximum speed, that is, maximum striking force. Also, the hip toggle must be done over a very short distance, and once completed it must come back as rapidly as possible to the position it was in before the toggle. It should be a rapid back-and-forth movement.

If you execute the technique with a rotation movement, you have to start the displacement of the hip with a rotation movement from the starting position. The leg executing the technique must be bent and start to straighten before striking the target. But if you want powerful striking force, multiple choices for combination techniques, and rapid position displacement after completing the technique, you must use the hip-propulsion movement.

Extreme precision is required, as previously discussed, since the time required to straighten your leg is very brief. You must be aligned in such a way to allow your technique to strike your target during the toggling movement. It is more difficult when the first movement necessary to displace your right hip in Figure 1 is a propulsion movement from the 6 o'clock position to the 1 o'clock position. From that point, the hip movement will be a toggle aided by the hip of the supporting left leg, which will bring the upper right hip from 1 o'clock to 12 o'clock. All this requires much concentration and mastery, but with practice you will succeed, and the benefits are largely worth the effort.

Returning to the last question: Can we propel the right hip to the 2 o'clock position and toggle both hips to displace the right hip to the 1 o'clock position? Once the right hip is propelled from the 6 o'clock position to the point facing 1 o'clock, your center of gravity is constantly changing. This is the desired outcome, since we learned that to initiate movement your center of gravity must change. If, for example, you weigh 220 pounds and are standing upright with your legs slightly spread apart, each leg supports a weight of 110 pounds. If you want to walk, there is a constant weight transfer from one leg to the other. Part of the weight is displaced forward, forcing you to move forward and consequently to walk. The weight is projected forward, and the faster you walk, as in running, the further forward the weight is projected.

In executing a *Bichagi*, more weight is transferred to the striking foot, according to the equation **striking force = mass × speed**. The more the mass increases, the greater the striking force. From this fact, the less weight that the supporting leg has to support, the faster the position displacement is, and therefore less energy is required. The maximum possible mass transfer on the striking leg is achieved once the hip is propelled further forward, when it has attained the 1 o'clock position, just before the toggling movement begins. At this point the hip has reached the point where it is most unstable or unbalanced; from what we just learned, we can develop greater speed by acquiring balance. Now we have high speed with a large mass. From the equation **striking force = mass × speed**, a large mass multiplied by high speed will produce a very powerful striking force. This represents the point when balance is most unstable and when the supporting leg has the least weight to support. This is when the toggling movement is most easily executed. So this answers the last question, in part, because we have learned the "why" – but not yet the "why not."

HYBRID *BICHAGI*

Before starting to describe the hybrid *Bichagi*, attention must be given to how superior the striking force of the hip-propulsion technique is compared to the hip-rotation technique. When the equation **striking force = mass × speed** is rearranged to put the emphasis on speed, we arrive at the formula **speed = striking**

force ÷ mass. For the student of taekwondo, both striking force and speed are very important. I would even say that up to a certain level, speed is more important than striking force.

Once you master the hip-propulsion movement, you can emphasize speed instead of force, because at this level the striking force that you develop is extreme. In the previous section I put much emphasis on the fact that by decreasing the mass transferred at the striking point we can increase speed, due to the fact that speed is inversely proportional to mass. But is there a way to decrease the mass transferred at the striking point? Yes, there is: When the right hip in Figure 1 is facing 6 o'clock and starts to be propelled forward, you will notice that until then, the hip is facing approximately 2:20. The center of gravity is too far behind pivot point 1. Trying to execute a technique before this point is useless, because you have neither a sufficiently solid foothold as a base nor sufficient forward projection to support a strong attack.

Anyone who has fired a rifle knows that strong shoulder support is necessary. If it is a high-caliber rifle and you pull the trigger without having properly braced it against your shoulder, the bullet leaving the barrel has a strong opposing force that will push the gun back strongly to hit your shoulder. The same principle applies if you try to execute a *Bichagi* with your hip in Figure 1 facing the 2:20 clock position. You would probably lose balance backward, which would allow your opponent to counterattack. But why not start to toggle the hip when it's facing 2 o'clock? We learned why we initiate the toggle at the 1 o'clock position, but we haven't learned why we don't start it at 2 o'clock.

At the 2:20 position, your center of gravity starts to transfer some mass toward your opponent, but not enough. At the 2 o'clock position, things become more interesting: your center of gravity is sufficiently forward to offer a solid base for good mass projection, allowing you to execute the technique. One advantage not yet discussed is the relative mass of the striking foot when the right hip is facing the 2 o'clock position. This relative mass is far smaller than when the hip is facing 1 o'clock. We are able to decrease the projected mass in the equation **speed = striking force ÷ mass**. Therefore, we can increase the speed of execution considerably.

In Figure 1, the opponent is in combat position at 12 o'clock. If the technique is completed once the right hip has reached the 1 o'clock position, the target will never be reached. To be able to move more than 1 hour on the clock would require a hip-rotation movement. This answers the question of why we can't propel the right hip to the 2 o'clock position and toggle both hips to displace the right hip to 1 o'clock. It is also possible to correct this weakness. While the hip is propelled to the 2 o'clock position, the knee must be aligned toward the opponent at 12 o'clock. The knee alignment can then correct the error caused by our position with respect to the target.

Also, to correct the other weakness of the vertical instead of horizontal striking force vector, you must perform a slight internal rotation of the leg, similar to the Charleston dance, with respect to right hip in Figure 1. This corrects the striking angle.

With the hybrid *Bichagi*, I have developed a technique that creates a very powerful striking force through the propulsion movement. By decreasing the relative mass, which increases the speed, it offers the potential advantage of redirecting the attack at will and offers a huge number of potential combination techniques that would otherwise be very difficult to perform. By working with a smaller mass, the practitioner's movement on the floor is more rapid after delivering the technique.

Think of a thin sheet of paper. Without considering the material's resistance, take a hammer, which has a large mass, and try to rip through the paper when it is being held by either side. The hammer will tear through it very easily. If the sheet of paper is held by only one hand, this task is impossible. Yet a single flick of the finger can easily rip through the paper when it is held by two hands. A finger has a much smaller mass than a hammer. Can speed inflict more damage than mass? Imagine using the same heavy hammer with the same movement to break a window. It is quite easy to break it into thousands of pieces. Imagine trying to break the same window with a flick of the finger. Clearly, in certain cases high speed is preferable, and in other cases large mass is essential.

The sheet of paper succeeds in neutralizing, or rather converting, the energy of the mass into movement. Because the paper can move rapidly, it can synchronize itself with the hammer's movement, converting its energy into movement and neutralizing the hammer's effect. The student of taekwondo can learn this in the "Synchronization" section in the "Basic Principles" chapter. The more a technique's striking force is developed by speed and not by mass, the more difficulty the opponent will have converting the energy into movement to neutralize its effect. If the force is developed using mass rather than speed, however, it is relatively simple to convert it into movement. Force developed this way will tend to displace the target instead of going through it.

The more a technique's striking force is developed by speed and not by mass, the more difficulty the opponent will have converting the energy into movement to neutralize its effect.

Fundamental Techniques

Fundamental taekwondo techniques performed with the hip-propulsion movement rather than the conventional hip-rotation movement are explained below, based on Figure 1 in the "Hip Movement" chapter above. The pictures depict techniques executed at full speed but with the striking range controlled. (Therefore, the center of gravity and thus more weight is on the standing leg in these pictures than you would find in regular practice. This was simply necessary in order to take the pictures.) My partner in these pictures is my wife, Nicole.

- **BICHAGI**

- **DOLRYA CHAGI**

- **YUP CHAGI**

- **DWI CHAGI**

- **MIL A CHAGI**

- **AHP CHAGI**

- **AHP BAHL HURIGI**

- **DWI DOLRYA CHAGI**

- **NEHRYUH CHAGI**

- **MOMTONG CHIRUGI**

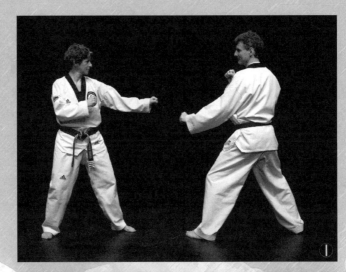

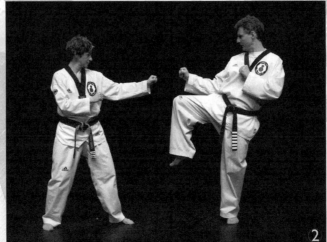

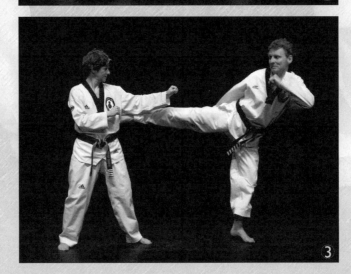

BICHAGI

(Angle-round Kick)

COMBAT POSITION WITH THE LEFT LEG IN FRONT:

Assume a position with the left leg pointing to 12 o'clock to execute a *Bichagi*. From pivot point 1, displace your right hip from 6 o'clock to 1 o'clock using the hip-propulsion movement, turning counterclockwise. At this point, your knee is bent, and your toes point to the floor. Straighten your knee, executing the *Bichagi*, while your hip toggles from 1 o'clock to 12 o'clock. This toggling movement is aided by the supporting left hip. Once the 12 o'clock position is reached, the technique is complete. The strike is delivered with the top of the foot.

COMBAT POSITION WITH THE RIGHT LEG IN FRONT:

Assume a position with the right leg pointing to 12 o'clock to execute a *Bichagi*. From pivot point 1, displace your left hip from 6 o'clock to 11 o'clock using the hip-propulsion movement, turning clockwise. At this point, your knee is bent, and your toes point to the floor. Straighten your knee, executing the *Bichagi*, while your hip toggles from 11 o'clock to 12 o'clock. This toggling movement is aided by the supporting right hip. Once the 12 o'clock position is reached, the technique is complete. The strike is delivered with the top of the foot.

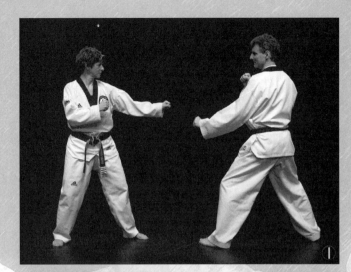

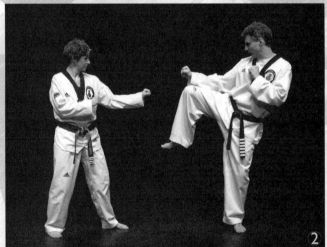

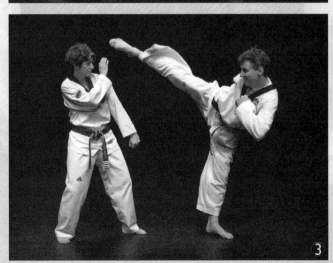

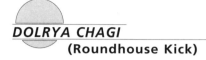

DOLRYA CHAGI
(Roundhouse Kick)

COMBAT POSITION WITH THE LEFT LEG IN FRONT:

Assume a position with the left leg pointing to 12 o'clock to execute a Roundhouse Kick. From pivot point 1, displace your right hip from 6 o'clock to 1 o'clock using the hip-propulsion movement, turning counterclockwise. The knee is high and bent, pointing upward and slightly pulls the hip upward, toes pointing to the floor. Straighten your knee, executing the *Dolrya Chagi*, while your hip toggles from 1 o'clock 12 o'clock. This toggling movement is aided by the supporting left hip. Once the 12 o'clock position is reached, the technique is complete. The strike is delivered with the top of the foot.

COMBAT POSITION WITH THE RIGHT LEG IN FRONT:

Assume a position with the right leg pointing to 12 o'clock to execute a Roundhouse Kick. From pivot point 1, displace your left hip from 6 o'clock to 11 o'clock using the hip-propulsion movement, turning clockwise. The knee is high and bent, pointing upward, and slightly pulls the hip upward, toes pointing to the floor. Straighten your knee, executing the *Dolrya Chagi*, while your hip toggles from 11 o'clock to 12 o'clock. This toggling movement is aided by the supporting right hip. Once the 12 o'clock position is reached, the technique is complete. The strike is delivered with the top of the foot.

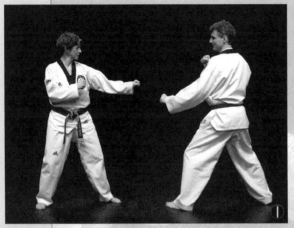

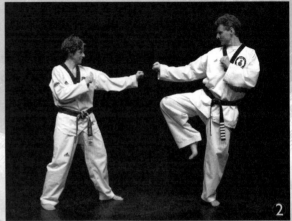

(to body)

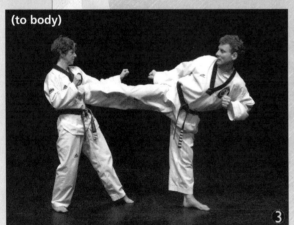

(to face)

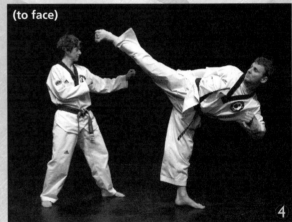

YUP CHAGI
(Side kick)

COMBAT POSITION WITH THE LEFT LEG IN FRONT:

Stand with your left leg pointing to 12 o'clock to execute a *Yup Chagi*. From pivot point 1, displace your right hip from 6 o'clock toward 12 o'clock using the hip-propulsion movement, turning counterclockwise. At this point, the knee is bent, pointing forward, the toes point to the floor, and the sole of the foot is slightly touching the knee. Straighten your knee forward, executing the *Yup Chagi,* while your hip toggles from the 12 o'clock position to 11 o'clock. This toggling movement is aided by the supporting left hip. Once the 11 o'clock position is reached, the technique is complete. The strike is delivered with the lower side of the heel, toes lifted and pointing inward, delivering powerful striking force.

COMBAT POSITION WITH THE RIGHT LEG IN FRONT:

Stand with your right leg pointing to 12 o'clock to execute a *Yup Chagi*. From pivot point 1, displace your left hip from 6 o'clock toward 12 o'clock using the hip-propulsion movement, turning clockwise. At this point, the knee is bent, pointing forward, the toes point to the floor, and the sole of the foot is slightly touching the knee. Straighten your knee forward, executing the *Yup Chagi,* while your hip toggles from the 12 o'clock position to 1 o'clock. This toggling movement is aided by the supporting right hip. Once the 1 o'clock position is reached, the technique is complete. The strike is delivered with the lower side of the heel, toes lifted and pointing inward, delivering powerful striking force.

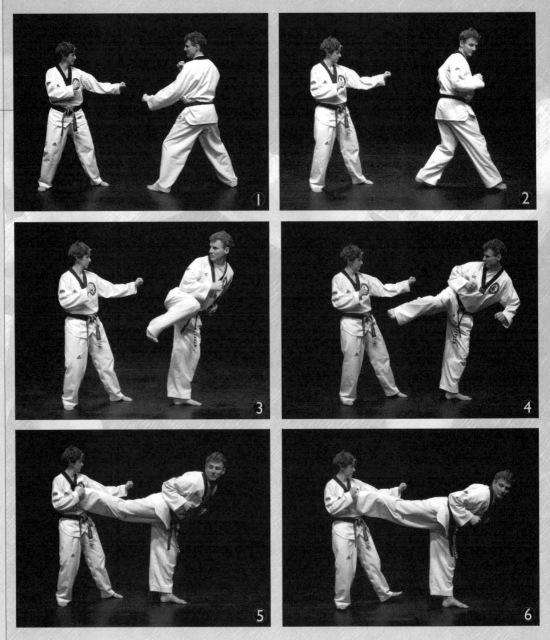

DWI CHAGI
(Back Kick)

COMBAT POSITION WITH THE LEFT LEG IN FRONT:

Stand with your left leg pointing to 12 o'clock to execute a *Dwi Chagi*. From pivot point 1, displace your right hip from pointing to 6 o'clock toward 11 o'clock using the hip-propulsion movement, turning clockwise. At this point, the knee is bent, pointing backward, and the toes point to the floor. Straighten your knee forward, executing the *Dwi Chagi*, while your hip toggles from the 11 o'clock position to 10 o'clock. This toggling movement is aided by the supporting left hip. Once the 10 o'clock position is reached, the technique is complete. The strike is delivered with the lower side of the heel, toes lifted and pointing inward, delivering powerful striking force.

COMBAT POSITION WITH THE RIGHT LEG IN FRONT:

Stand with your right leg pointing to 12 o'clock to execute a *Dwi Chagi*. From pivot point 1, displace your left hip from pointing to 6 o'clock toward 1 o'clock using the hip-propulsion movement, turning counterclockwise. At this point, the knee is bent, pointing backward, and the toes point to the floor. Straighten your knee forward, executing the *Dwi Chagi*, while your hip toggles from the 1 o'clock position to 2 o'clock. This toggling movement is aided by the supporting right hip. Once the 2 o'clock position is reached, the technique is complete. The strike is delivered with the lower side of the heel, toes lifted and pointing inward, delivering powerful striking force.

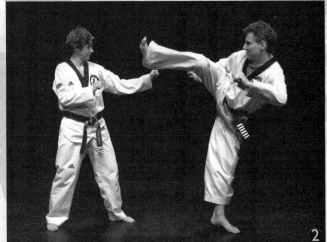

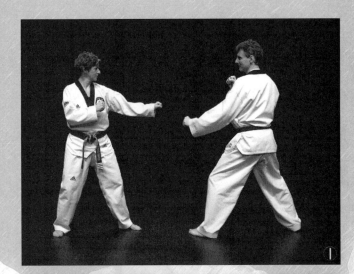

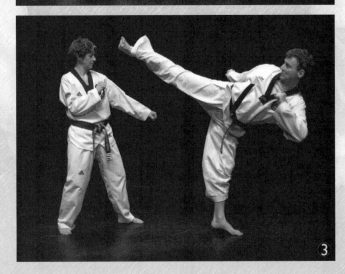

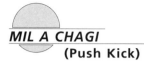

MIL A CHAGI
(Push Kick)

COMBAT POSITION WITH THE LEFT LEG IN FRONT:

Stand with your left leg pointing to 12 o'clock to execute a *Mil A Chagi*. From pivot point 1, displace your right hip from 6 o'clock toward 2 o'clock using the hip-propulsion movement, turning counterclockwise. At this point, your knee is bent with your leg parallel to the floor, toes pointing toward 11 o'clock and bent inward. Straighten your knee forward, executing the *Mil A Chagi*, while your hip toggles from the 2 o'clock position to 1 o'clock. This toggling movement is aided by the supporting left hip. Once the 1 o'clock position is reached, the technique is complete. The strike is delivered with the sole of the foot, toes lifted and pointing inward, delivering a powerful striking force. Once the technique is complete, the toes point toward 10 o'clock.

COMBAT POSITION WITH THE RIGHT LEG IN FRONT:

Stand with your right leg pointing to 12 o'clock to execute a *Mil A Chagi*. From pivot point 1, displace your left hip from 6 o'clock toward 10 o'clock using the hip-propulsion movement, turning clockwise. At this point, your knee is bent with your leg parallel to the floor, toes pointing toward 1 o'clock and bent inward. Straighten your knee forward, executing the *Mil A Chagi*, while your hip toggles from the 10 o'clock position to 11 o'clock. This toggling movement is aided by the supporting right hip. Once the 11 o'clock position is reached, the technique is complete. The strike is delivered with the sole of the foot, toes lifted and pointing inward, delivering a powerful striking force. Once the technique is complete, the toes point toward 2 o'clock.

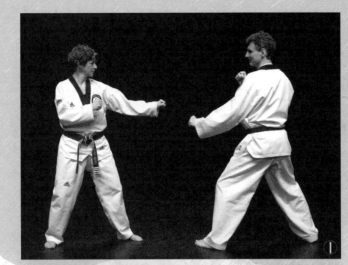

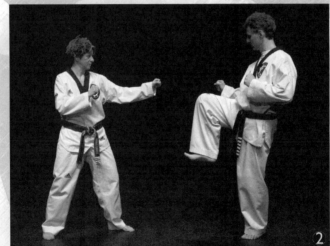

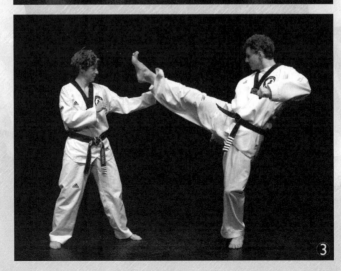

AHP CHAGI
(Front Kick)

COMBAT POSITION WITH THE LEFT LEG IN FRONT:

Stand with your left leg pointing to 12 o'clock to execute an *Ahp Chagi*. From pivot point 1, displace your right hip from 6 o'clock to 2 o'clock using the hip-propulsion movement, turning counter-clockwise. At this point, your knee is bent, pointing forward, and your toes point to the floor. Straighten your knee forward, executing the *Ahp Chagi*, while your hip toggles from 2 o'clock to 1 o'clock, pushing the knee. Your toes bend inward while your foot bends outward. This toggling movement is aided by the supporting left hip. Once the 1 o'clock position is reached, the technique is complete. The strike is delivered with the ball of the foot, toes lifted and pointing inward, delivering powerful striking force.

COMBAT POSITION WITH THE RIGHT LEG IN FRONT:

Stand with your right leg pointing to 12 o'clock to execute an *Ahp Chagi*. From pivot point 1, displace your left hip from 6 o'clock to 10 o'clock using the hip-propulsion movement, turning clockwise. At this point, your knee is bent, pointing forward, and your toes point to the floor. Straighten your knee forward, executing the *Ahp Chagi*, while your hip toggles from 10 o'clock to 11 o'clock, pushing the knee. Your toes bend inward while your foot bends outward. This toggling movement is aided by the supporting right hip. Once the 11 o'clock position is reached, the technique is complete. The strike is delivered with the ball of the foot, toes lifted and pointing inward, delivering powerful striking force.

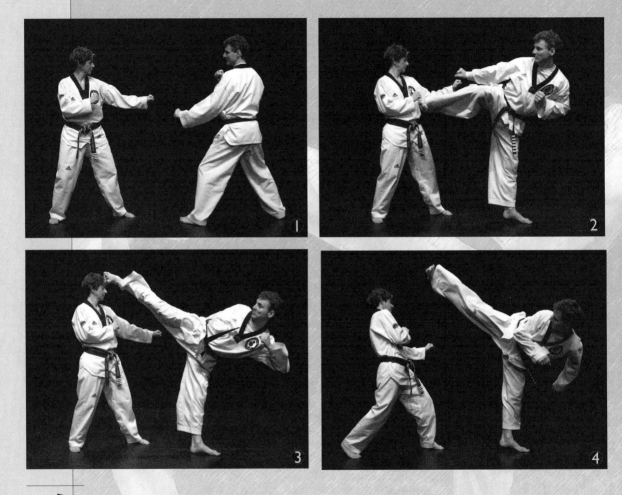

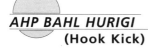

AHP BAHL HURIGI
(Hook Kick)

COMBAT POSITION WITH THE LEFT LEG IN FRONT:

Stand with your left leg pointing to 12 o'clock to execute an *Ahp Bahl Hurigi.* From pivot point 1, displace your right hip from 6 o'clock to 12 o'clock using the hip-propulsion movement, turning counterclockwise. Your body is bent slightly forward to bring your knee in closer to your chest, your leg parallel to the floor, foot horizontal. Straighten your knee forward, bringing your foot close to the 12 o'clock position. In this position, your heel is close to the side of the target, and your body tends to be at 45 degrees to the knee. Your hip toggles from 12 o'clock to 11 o'clock while your body is straightened to 180 degrees to the knee, which is now fully extended. Your leg travels on a horizontal plane, completely extended during the toggling movement.

Once the target is struck, the leg is retracted by bending the knee while the hip toggles back to its initial position at 12 o'clock. You are now ready to assume the combat position. If you do not toggle your hip, your leg will make a circular movement. Take a close look at figures 6 and 7 on page 60.

COMBAT POSITION WITH THE RIGHT LEG IN FRONT:

Stand with your right leg pointing to 12 o'clock to execute an *Ahp Bahl Hurigi.* From pivot point 1, displace your left hip from 6 o'clock to 12 o'clock using the hip-propulsion movement, turning clockwise. Your body will be bent slightly forward to bring your knee in closer to your chest, your leg parallel to the floor, foot horizontal. Straighten your knee forward, bringing your foot close to the 12 o'clock position. In this position, your heel is close to the side of the target, and your body tends to be at 45 degrees to the knee. Your hip toggles from 12 o'clock to 1 o'clock while your body is straightened to 180 degrees to the knee, which is now fully extended. Your leg travels on a horizontal plane, completely extended during the toggling movement.

Once the target is struck, the leg is retracted by bending the knee while the hip toggles back to its initial position at 12 o'clock. You are now ready to assume the combat position. If you do not toggle your hip, your leg will make a circular movement. Take a close look at figures 6 and 7 on page 60.

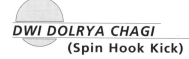

DWI DOLRYA CHAGI
(Spin Hook Kick)

COMBAT POSITION WITH THE LEFT LEG IN FRONT:

Stand with your left leg pointing to 12 o'clock to execute a *Dwi Dolrya Chagi*. From pivot point 1, displace your right hip from 6 o'clock to 12 o'clock using the hip-propulsion movement, turning clockwise. With an initial impetus, your upper body will develop sufficient energy to rotate 360 degrees. This movement is aided by your arms serving as levers. Your body is bent slightly forward to bring your knee closer to your chest, your leg parallel to the floor, foot horizontal. Your head rapidly turns clockwise toward 12 o'clock. Once your hip has reached 12 o'clock, straighten your knee forward to 12 o'clock, bringing your foot close to 12 o'clock. In this position, your heel is close to the side of the target, and your body tends to be at 45 degrees to the knee. Your hip toggles from 12 o'clock to 11 o'clock while your body straightens 180 degrees to the knee, which is now fully extended. Your leg travels on a horizontal plane, completely extended during the toggling movement.

Once the target is struck, your leg is bent in such a way as to increase hip control. The energy developed by your shoulders will tend to terminate the 360-degree rotation that the body has completed. If you do not toggle your hip, your leg will make a circular movement (see Figure 6).

Notice in Figure 6 that with a *Dwi Dolrya Chagi*, the impact on the target is maintained during the time between point H and point I. An opponent receiving such a kick can easily move to transform the energy developed by this technique. But if you use the propulsion technique to bring your hip to a position where a toggling

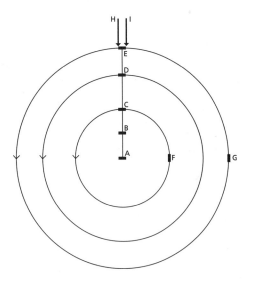

figure 6 : Range of striking with
a hip rotation movement

figure 7 : Range of striking with a
hip-propulsion movement

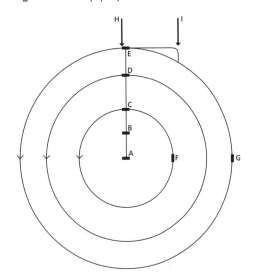

movement is possible, the striking range of your kicking leg is considerably increased. This will allow you to maintain your impact energy for a longer time, between point H and point I, leaving your opponent with practically no chance to transform that energy into movement (see Figure 7).

Once the target is struck, you can easily retract your hip to stop the 360-degree rotation of the upper body that the shoulders initiated and return to its initial position, ready to combine rapidly with other techniques. Once your hip has toggled to the 11 o'clock position, you can choose to come back to the initial starting point rather than retracting it, but this time counterclockwise. This choice can dramatically change the combat dynamics by giving you the option of returning your kicking leg to its initial starting place at 6 o'clock to be able to use a second attack technique rapidly. The strike of the *Dwi Dolrya Chagi* is delivered with the back part of the heel, the foot horizontal, delivering very powerful striking force.

COMBAT POSITION
WITH THE RIGHT LEG IN FRONT:

Stand with your right leg pointing to 12 o'clock to execute a *Dwi Dolrya Chagi*. From pivot point 1, displace your left hip from 6 o'clock to 12 o'clock using the hip-propulsion movement, turning counterclockwise. With an initial impetus, your upper body will develop sufficient energy to rotate 360 degrees. This movement is aided by your arms serving as levers. Your body is bent slightly forward to bring your knee closer to your chest, your leg parallel to the floor, foot horizontal. Your head rapidly turns counterclockwise toward 12 o'clock. Once your hip has reached 12 o'clock, straighten your knee forward to 12 o'clock, bringing your foot close to 12 o'clock. In this position, your heel is close to the side of the target, and your body tends to be at 45 degrees to the knee. Your hip toggles from 12 o'clock to 1 o'clock while your body straightens 180 degrees to the knee, which is now fully extended. Your leg travels on a horizontal plane completely extended during the toggling movement.

Once the target is struck, you can easily retract your hip to stop the 360-degree rotation of the upper body that the shoulders initiated and return to the initial position, ready to combine rapidly with other techniques. Once your hip has toggled to the 11 o'clock position, you can choose to come back to the initial starting point rather than retracting it. This time, use a counter-clockwise motion to bring it back to 6 o'clock, which will allow you to use a second clockwise technique right away – surprising your opponent. The strike of the *Dwi Dolrya Chagi* is delivered with the back part of the heel, the foot horizontal, delivering very powerful striking force.

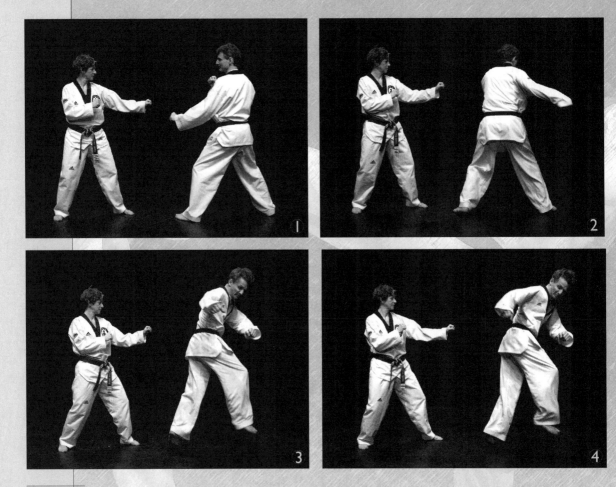

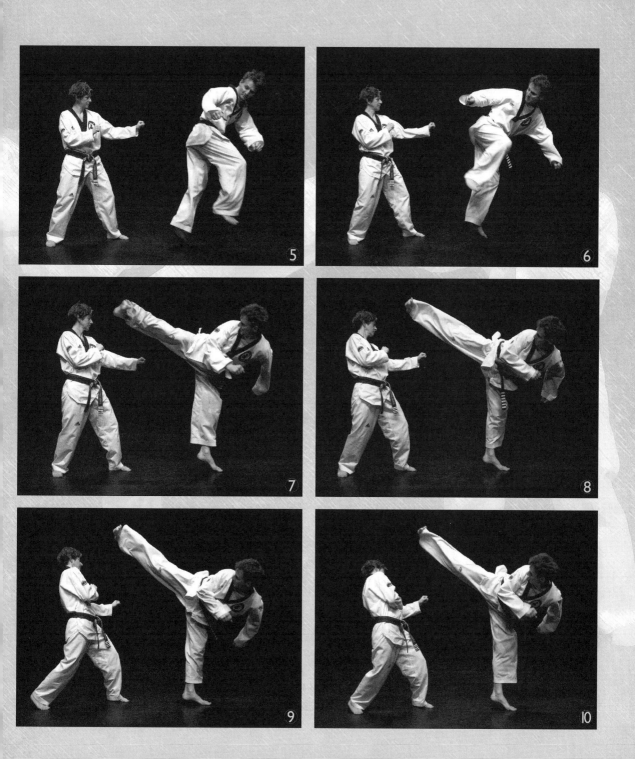

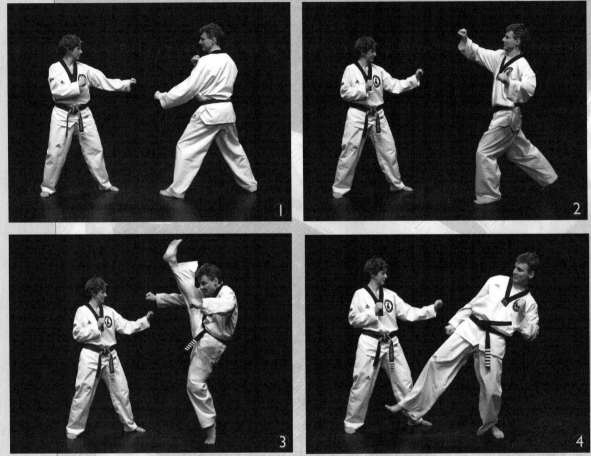

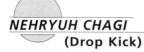

NEHRYUH CHAGI
(Drop Kick)

COMBAT POSITION WITH THE LEFT LEG IN FRONT:

Stand with your left leg pointing to 12 o'clock to execute a *Nehryuh Chagi*. From pivot point 1, displace your right hip from 6 o'clock toward 2 o'clock using the hip-propulsion movement, turning counterclockwise. At this point, your knee is bent and moving upward. Straighten your knee before your hip toggles from 2 o'clock to 1 o'clock, slightly lowering your center of gravity. This toggling movement is aided by the supporting left leg. The leg strikes downward to hit the target during the toggling movement in executing the *Nehryuh Chagi*. The strike is delivered with the heel.

COMBAT POSITION WITH THE RIGHT LEG IN FRONT:

Stand with your right leg pointing to 12 o'clock to execute a *Nehryuh Chagi*. From pivot point 1, displace your left hip from 6 o'clock toward 10 o'clock using the hip-propulsion movement, turning clockwise. At this point, your knee is bent and moving upward. Straighten your knee before your hip toggles from 10 o'clock to 11 o'clock, slightly lowering your center of gravity. This toggling movement is aided by the supporting right leg. The leg strikes downward to hit the target during the toggling movement in executing the *Nehryuh Chagi*. The strike is delivered with the heel.

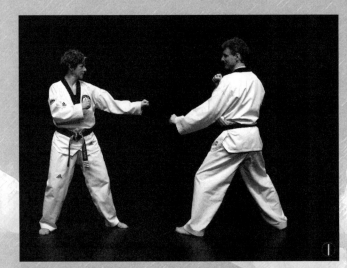

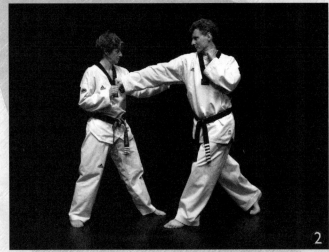

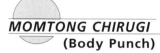

MOMTONG CHIRUGI
(Body Punch)

COMBAT POSITION WITH THE LEFT LEG IN FRONT:

With your left leg forward, your right hip is propelled forward with the same impetus as in the *Bichagi* technique. Your rear foot stays back on the floor, but to help the hip displacement, the heel is lifted to extend the hip movement. Your right shoulder, synchronized with your right hip, projects your right fist forward. Meanwhile, your left shoulder is retracted to permit the right shoulder to displace toward the target. All these movement are executed like a wave of energy that starts from the abdomen, moves toward the shoulders, and then to the fist. Your fist contracts at the impact; this is done with the joints of the index and middle fingers.

COMBAT POSITION WITH THE RIGHT LEG IN FRONT:

With your right leg forward, your left hip is propelled forward with the same impetus as in the *Bichagi* technique. Your rear foot stays back on the floor, but to help the hip displacement, the heel is lifted to extend the hip movement. Your left shoulder, synchronized with your left hip, projects your left fist forward. Meanwhile, your right shoulder is retracted to permit the left shoulder to displace toward the target. All these movement are executed like a wave of energy that starts from the abdomen, moves toward the shoulders, and then to the fist. Your fist contracts at the impact; this is done with the joints of the index and middle fingers.

Sparring

Depending on their character, certain people are better in defensive positions while others perform best in offensive positions. We must train for both, because in sparring, even if we start in a defensive position, we need to change to an offensive position when required.

It is important to know which position corresponds to our character so that we can better control the match to favor our best position. Many practitioners prefer to maintain a defensive position even if the best position for them is an offensive one. The reason is simple: reaction time is shorter than action time. This means that if you are well trained and assume a proper defensive position, once your opponent initiates an attack, you have time to counterattack. But if the best position for your character is offensive, there is a greater likelihood that in assuming a defensive position with an experienced opponent, your reaction time to counterattack will be greater than your opponent's action time. In the "Visualization" chapter I describe a technique that allows the conversion of a reaction into an action. This allows us to maintain the position that is best suited to our character.

The taekwondo blocking techniques become more synchronization techniques that, once mastered, permit you to convert each opponent's attack into a counterattack without using any blocks. When you completely understand the true meaning of synchronization, you can more easily anticipate attacks from your opponent. Your arms are used as a tool to protect your body, but using synchronization you can convert the energy of your opponent's attack into a movement. During this movement's execution, your center of gravity will be displaced in such a way to allow the execution of a counterattack. The result is that when your opponent attacks, you receive the technique by protecting yourself with your arms while moving your center of gravity to synchronize it to your opponent's technique, placing you in a position that allows you to deliver a counterattack.

Here I must clarify what "receive" means. Imagine walking on a sidewalk when suddenly you notice an object falling from the roof of a building above your head. Your natural reflex is to raise your arms to protect yourself and move out of the object's path. In sparring the response should be similar, but you must move *closer* to your opponent to allow you safely to make a rapid and efficient counterattack. In taekwondo we develop this natural reflex to produce efficient counterattacks in sparring.

Many martial arts do not practice displacement techniques. In my opinion, displacement techniques are both important and efficient. They are a natural reaction that our reflexes know how to perform. We must exploit this reflex to our advantage.

There is a risk to remaining in the trajectory of a strike and simply attempting to block it. As an example, imagine walking on a railroad track and suddenly hearing a train coming at full speed behind you. Would you remain in its path and try to block the train with your arm? Surely not; logically you would move out of the way. A similar situation occurs on a smaller scale during sparring when you face an opponent executing a powerful kick technique toward you. Would it be logical to remain in place and attempt to block his foot technique with your arm? Imagine the energy your arm would receive from that leg. Even if you succeeded in blocking it, it is a strike to a vital part of your body. The logical response is to move out of its path and thereby change its trajectory. As we learn in physics, energy is neither created nor destroyed. This means that the energy delivered by your opponent's technique has to be absorbed by your blocking technique that tries to stop it.

We must offer the least resistance to the opponent's attack to minimize its destructive force. It is difficult to break through a sheet of paper with your finger when the sheet is held by only one side. But if it is held at both sides, the task becomes easy. This applies in taekwondo as a technique that relates to the term *receive*. We cannot create nor destroy energy, but we can transform it. Considering this law, in taekwondo we have developed techniques to transform an opponent's attack into a positive movement. The goal is to synchronize our speed to the opponent's speed so that the striking force is decreased to the point that it is practically completely neutralized.

Imagine jumping out of a train traveling at sixty miles per hour. Your fall would be violent. Instead, if another train were traveling at the same speed parallel to your train and in the same direction, and you were to jump on it, your fall would not be as damaging. The difference here is synchronization.

The maximum force delivered in a taekwondo technique can cover an average distance of four inches. This means that with good synchronization, the displacement distance required to receive an attack with a minimum of pain is very short.

To permit synchronization, we must develop our coordination to the maximum, learn how to judge distances, and be able to determine the direction, range, and speed of an attack in a fraction of a second. This will help you receive an opponent's attack and allow you to execute a counterattack technique while your opponent is executing an attack technique.

Mind

We must keep an open mind to detect openings where we can attack or counterattack with the most efficient technique at the precise optimal moment.

Sparring situations are unpredictable, which reinforces why we must practice attacks and counterattacks for a variety of different situations. We must not let our minds be inhibited. This happens when we train our brains for a specific situation without practicing its flexibility or logic. If you condition your brain to react in a specific way when faced with a particular situation, your mind cannot adapt if that situation suddenly changes for the worse, and you may react in the wrong way.

As an example, imagine living in a house with two doors. The back door has a doorbell that makes a single chime, while the front door has a doorbell that makes a double chime. The difference in the sounds is so that you can distinguish where your visitor is standing. As soon as your brain receives the signal of a double chime, it gives you the instruction to answer the front door. But what would happen if the front doorbell broke and chimed only once when it was activated? If a visitor rings the front doorbell, the brain hears one chime and gives the instruction to answer the back door. When you open the back door you find no one there. It is not the brain's error; it was *trained* to react this way.

In this example, no lives were in danger. But what would happen with such training in a sparring competition? This is where the importance of a good training program, one that prepares us for all possible situations, comes in. Such training is imperative in taekwondo.

This is also why many times even high-level taekwondo champions feel powerless when they get involved in a street fight. It happens when students train using a limited or insufficient variety of attack techniques. If you are attacked on the street, and if the attack technique is not one that the brain was trained to react to, how to react will temporarily be unclear. The reaction time to send instructions to the muscles to counterattack will be longer.

Imagine playing tic-tac-toe on a computer, and the programmer forgot to include one possible move in the software. The computer will be able to play the game, but if you place an X in the square that the programmer forgot to account for, the computer will not know what to do. The game will either freeze or give an error message, allowing you to win the game.

Taekwondo training must prepare the brain for all possibilities to allow for a proper defense when faced with any situation. We must condition ourselves to decide rapidly what action is required when we are faced with different attacks. We must not create any limits, because as a whole the mind does not have any limits. We must understand a counterattack before applying it. In sparring it is the brain that gives instruction to the muscles. Therefore, we

For any situation that you choose to imagine, the brain can order the body to react as if the situation were real.

must prepare the brain properly. Taekwondo was developed for this purpose.

The mind does not differentiate between the imaginary and the real. For any situation that you choose to imagine, the brain can order the body to react as if the situation were real. We have all heard the saying that we are responsible for our own misfortunes. If we imagine ourselves as losers, then there is a good chance that we will become losers. On the other hand, if we imagine ourselves as winners, we significantly increase the chance of becoming one.

If you've ever seen a magician or illusionist perform, how many moves was he or she able to make that you could not see?

With agile fingers, but also following a rhythm and with excellent synchronization, the magician succeeds in drawing your attention to a less significant action, thereby performing a more important action without it being noticed. In other words, he is able to make you look where he wants you to look to outsmart you. In taekwondo, this process is called a feint. It is a way to hide your real intentions to outsmart your opponent.

We must master the feint techniques. Your opponent is outsmarted, preparing for a simulated attack and moving into a favorable position for the real attack. Feints are useful to create openings in your opponent's defenses. In executing them, you must pay careful attention to your opponent for two main reasons:

1. **During the feint's execution, you must constantly search for an opening in the opponent's defenses to allow an efficient attack technique.**

2. **During the feint's execution, you must stay alert and on the defensive because the opponent can attack during that time. This is especially true if the opponent judges your defenses to be weak, or simply realizes the true nature of the feint.**

To be effective, a feint must be executed in such a way that the opponent believes you really have the intention to attack with a specific technique. If he or she detects hesitation on your part or a lack of conviction in the feint's execution, the technique will be revealed as only a feint, and the result could be disastrous.

During its execution, your concentration level must be extremely high because you can never be completely certain of what your opponent's reaction to your feint will be. If your reaction time is too long once the opening in your opponent's defenses is obvious, your opponent will have the opportunity to attack. Your level of consciousness during that delay elevates your mind to a state of questioning. In that frame of mind your reaction time is even greater because it is an intellectual state of mind, as explained in the "Visualization" chapter.

Combinations

In sparring, your opponent is not often in a position to simplify your attack. If you are well matched, your opponent should know how to correctly protect him – or herself. This is why, in many cases, the first attack you execute does not reach its intended target with the expected force. This also demonstrates the necessity of a second technique immediately following the first to act as its complement. The first technique will serve to put your opponent in a desirable position to allow your second technique to reach its target.

This principle is the same as in a chess game: you move your pawns with the goal of provoking a move by your opponent that will lead to a checkmate. You must have a combat strategy or plan and play to force your opponent into check.

This is not as simple as it sounds. The obvious danger of combinations is that at a certain point, your back may be turned toward your opponent, who could take advantage of that moment of vulnerability to attack. But if your combination technique is performed adequately and rapidly, such opportunities should not exist because you are prepared to attack with your second technique.

While training, it is therefore important to execute combinations rapidly and with fluidity so that your balance is not affected. A failure in speed and fluidity creates another opportunity for your opponent to attack. Everything must be synchronized to allow the execution of combinations at high speed while maintaining good balance and good synchronization at all times without losing striking force.

Positive Thinking

You must drive negative thoughts from your mind. Wake up each morning being happy for the new day. This will help fill you with energy.

As athletes, we are always searching for ways to economize and increase our energy reserves. Positive thinking is an excellent way to achieve this goal. For skeptics, I have a story to convince you of this.

Imagine that you are head over heels in love and everything seems beautiful. You're living on love. One morning, you wake up in a great mood, and the telephone rings. It is your lover, who announces that everything is over between you. What a disaster! All of your energy has just vanished, and your arms drop. You have not expended any physical effort that required energy, but still, you feel exhausted. For every action there is a reaction. A negative thought generates a negative reaction within the body. A positive thought therefore generates a positive reaction within the body. As the saying goes, after a storm comes a calm. Even if you face a negative situation, you must take it on positively to be able to adequately refocus your energy. You must see the good side of things to avoid mental exhaustion.

Everyone is free to make choices. We must choose what is important to us and what touches us. Many people live in an illusion, not knowing how to recognize what is really going on. When I talk about positive thoughts, I do not mean to encourage you to live in an illusion when you're faced with a difficult situation. When we face a difficult situation, we must recognize the truth in it. We often give it the significance of something worse than it really is. In most cases, once we have gone through something that had originally appeared unbearable, we later realize that in reality it was not as terrible as anticipated.

Confrontations often appear much worse than they really are. We have a lot more strength than we realize. We must have confidence in our ability to handle it, and often our interpretation of the situation will limit our possibilities. For every situation, there is something positive that we can reach out for, no matter how frightening or disastrous it appears. Why think differently? If there is something we can do to change the situation, we don't have to worry about it; we just have to do it. Likewise, if there is nothing we can do about it, we don't have to worry about it because we cannot change it, except the way the situation affects us.

The eyes transmit images to the brain, but it is the mind that interprets them.

Here is a simple example. You are driving your car on the highway on your way to work. Everything is going well, the weather is nice, and the road conditions are excellent. You are right on schedule. Suddenly, you notice other cars in front of you are slowing down, to the point that the traffic is no longer moving. You realize that there is an accident ahead, that there are emergency vehicles. How will you react? Some people react with anger, aggression, or anxiety. Your heart rate accelerates, your blood pressure rises, and you begin to perspire, watching the time go by and knowing you will be late for work, imagining all kind of scenarios that amplify your anxiety. Once the highway is clear you continue on your way to work, but now you're late, exhausted, have a headache, and basically your whole day is ruined. There was nothing you could do for the people injured; the paramedics were already there. You couldn't do anything to clear the road and improve the traffic flow. Why did you feel such anxiety?

Other people react differently, and the situation does not seem so dramatic. You soon realize that you cannot do anything to change the traffic conditions. You accept it and take out your briefcase to get started on your work. Or you might read, listen to music, or practice visualization techniques to relax and help you get through your work day or other activities. Once you arrive at work, you are full of energy and ready to take on the workday. You have dealt positively with a situation that to someone else would have appeared completely negative. You had the choice to sustain the negative or to act positively.

It is not always easy to find the positive. It is a reflex that you can develop, especially if you realize how much energy is drawn by the negative. Positive thoughts will make you feel better, and situations will begin to appear as not so dire. Remember that the eyes transmit images to the brain, but it is the mind that interprets them. So can you see the importance of appearances? I've also added another story in this book's conclusion on this topic.

Visualization

In this chapter, I want to present a visualization technique that will help you convert an attack into a counterattack. Specifically, with this technique it should be possible to execute an attack in the same amount of time as a counterattack.

Many stages of life give us the tools we need to help us attain enlightenment. I sincerely believe that taekwondo can be a wonderful tool to help us attain that objective. I often say, "I am a black belt," rather than, "I have a black belt." Being a black belt is the result of something that has developed within. In theory, when you have attained the red belt, you have developed many physical skills. Many hours of physical exercise were required to attain this level, and you are ready to seek more energy and more control using mental energy. On this path, you will seek a certain balance that, in return, will help you become a black belt. This requires a voyage within, the goal of which is self-discovery. You must develop your senses to be more aware and more sensitive to your surroundings.

Just because we know what a tree is does not mean that we understand the entire forest. Personalities, emotions, and facial gestures all have variations. So as not to get lost in these appearances, we must exercise our minds to perceive what our eyes alone cannot see. The forest won't look the same at all.

The term *taekwondo* signifies the art of the foot strike *(tae)* and the punch *(kwon)*. This is the physical side. More important is the *do*, which signifies the way of life on the philosophical side. Reading this book, you'll notice a key word: *sincerity*. In reality, my teaching is founded on this word. You'll understand the importance of this word a little later in this chapter.

Most taekwondo techniques were developed thousands of years ago by studying how wild animals fought each other. Nature protects itself, and the closer we get to nature, the more we can feel the force of life. Nature has much to teach that cannot be expressed in words. It is surprising how much energy you can recover by immersing yourself in it.

As a taekwondo instructor, I know that practitioners must be trained to the height of their physical and mental abilities. As in many sports, there are scientific methods to develop endurance, flexibility, striking force, and precision. Diet is a factor to be included among them. These scientific methods improve daily, mainly because of the Olympics, which encourage people to study ways to develop the best possible athletes. A good trainer is taught to offer follow-up to a practitioner. The *do* side of taekwondo is less known but may help change the way we spar and the way we live.

One of my students, Simonne – age fifty-three when she registered – saw a taekwondo demonstration that my wife and I were performing on television. She was impressed by our movements. We were sparring and using force, speed, and precision, but with gentleness and respect in our eyes. After the program I gave an interview in which many people noticed my deep sincerity, and I soon had an increase in students, among them Simonne. Now in her seventies, she is a second-dan black belt and teaches taekwondo to children and adults under my supervision. She says, "Taekwondo is like a love story." It is like a love story because when we are sincere with ourselves, we can be sincere with others, and this brings warmth to our hearts because it is nature's way.

Many people wear masks. These masks can help us get through certain obstacles that life puts in our path. But we have to know that wearing a mask makes the next step more difficult. If we want to grow, we must remove the mask to face life's next steps. Eventually all the masks must disappear, and while that may make it difficult to look in a mirror, if these masks have been worn for a long period of time there is a high probability that the face reflected in the mirror will be unknown to us. When we are younger, we have very little life experience. It is understandable that we feel the need to wear a mask to feel secure going through life's early stages. As we grow older, we gain sufficient self-confidence to be strong enough to let the mask drop and go through life's stages with our own identity.

One of the objectives I had when I wrote this book was to create a tool that I could give to the parents of my students to help them understand what is being taught. Students are taught to throw kicks, perform in competitions, and defend themselves.

Most importantly, they must discover their own identity, develop self-confidence, and be loyal and respectful. In return, they will be respected by others. I do my best to give them the best tools available to discover their own well-balanced philosophy of life. The black-belt students feel the force that pushes them to seek out the balance that is so essential in life. My role, then, is as a guide, where the effort and work must come from the heart and all masks are dropped, showing our true nature.

Before starting taekwondo training, many students have the tendency to believe that once the black-belt level is attained, there is nothing more to learn. After forty years of martial arts training, I would say rather that the black-belt level leads us to realize how small we are in the universe, just a tiny part of all the different known and unknown forces ruling life. Thinking that we're omniscient is the most obvious mistake that hinders our growth.

How can we seek enlightenment if we don't know ourselves? As a black-belt student, you must develop respect for your surroundings if you want to grow. You must be aware that sincerity is important and that it will help you to drop all the masks. Your true nature will reveal itself, and the learning process will continue. With sincerity, the heart will let the mind see what the eyes alone could not see before. With sincerity, the heart will allow the mind to understand what it could not before.

I have seen so many changes in my students. In her seventies, Simonne learned how to defend herself. She even came to assist me in giving demonstrations, breaking wooden boards with her techniques. She participated in a Pumsae competition, and although she did not win, the event itself provided a challenge that

Perfection closes the door to learning.

helped her grow further, a challenge she needed. Even though she did not win, she also did not lose, because she won the challenge of the fight against herself, which made her stronger – and this is taekwondo. Taekwondo gives us the tools to place ourselves in situations where we are challenged to be stronger and live life as it should be lived.

To clarify the belt color system, we must set small, realizable objectives. When a color has been acquired, we gain confidence and self-realization. We are then ready for the next objective.

Everyday life is full of stress. At work, we have to meet deadlines that are always getting shorter, our workload may become heavy, and then we easily get exhausted. We start to see only the mountains, forgetting that there are lovely valleys between them. It is easy to become exhausted when we only see mountains before us, when everything seems difficult to reach. We should be able to step back and gather energy while crossing the valleys. We must develop concentration to allow our minds to be oriented not to be disturbed by distractions that can waste energy. The same mental attitude applies in everyday life and during competition. We must not let ourselves be affected by our opponent in combat and feel defeated before the end of the competition. Until it is over, there is still a chance, and as long there is a chance, we must hang on to it. So many things are relative, and our perception of all situations depends on many factors. How can we see the truth without being influenced by these different disguises?

The eye is similar to a window. From inside a house, we can easily see sunlight through the window, but the window is not the light. Its role is only to let the light in. When we're driving on a rainy day, we can see through the windshield and drive safely. But if we look at the raindrops on the windshield, the image behind them becomes unclear, and we miss what we need to see to drive safely. Similarly, the mind must be trained to allow us to see what the eyes are trying to show us. As a student, when you are sincere, your heart helps you to bring your mind to a calm and serene state, which allows your eyes to offer the necessary vision and your mind to perceive what needs to be seen.

As you evolve as a black-belt student, you become more and more aware of the evolution of your state of mind and how calm you feel. Many things are then perceived in your surroundings that you were not aware of before. Walking in nature becomes marvelous and peaceful, and you start to feel the need for contemplation. Your evolution continues as you seek more enlightenment.

In order to master that state of mind, visualization can be an incredible tool. Since the brain does not differentiate between real and imaginary, visualization can be used for many different purposes.

Fear is often considered to be a lack of mental control over the imagination. When you are in a stressful situation that stimulates your metabolism, you can easily calm it through visualization. You can use your imagination. By projecting yourself, in your mind, to a beach covered with nice white sand, letting yourself enjoy the sun, listening to the waves along with the birds, your brain can come to a point where you can actually believe you are there. Your muscles then relax, and your heartbeat slows. For all this to happen, the beach image must appear as real as possible in your mind. Every little detail must be present, and all your senses must be activated. You must see yourself there and feel like you are there.

The performance of a taekwondo technique is enhanced when visualization techniques are used. We must train our minds to make our bodies feel the movement of the technique before we execute it. At first, we use our physical side to exercise our mind. As our abilities improve, mental exercises will be used to train our physical movements. In taekwondo, students train to be strong both physically and mentally. They seek the balance between these two energies, the physical and the mental, to reach perfect harmony.

Fire is a good example. It is a source of light, and light is energy. Fire is also a source of heat, and heat is energy. Heat and light are known to be two different sources of energy, but in fire one cannot exist without the other. At the dawn of humanity, the tribe that possessed fire as a tool had great power. The tribe that had not mastered it tried to steal it to protect the lives of its members. Nowadays, people can control fire, and so the quest for it has ended. We now seek tranquility and enlightenment. Similar to fire, we possess two different sources of energy: the physical and the mental. As with fire, one does not exist without the other. The problem in this modern era is that many people seek only to develop one and forget the importance of the other. When taekwondo training is well-balanced, both energies are developed. In giving a certain degree of balance to my students, I use visualization techniques in each of my courses.

Once they are adults, too many students try to intellectualize the techniques of taekwondo. This creates resistance in their movements. We must learn to let the movement flow like water, to follow the current instead of trying to swim against it. This philosophy applies in life as well as in taekwondo classes. Visualization will help you feel the techniques with your whole body instead of trying to intellectualize them. Intellectualization uses brain power that can prevent you from attaining speed, precision, striking force, and satori (enlightenment). Through visualization, you can command your brain to produce energy that will bring self-confidence along with a feeling of well-being. In combat, your opponent's movements will appear slower, giving you time to respond properly.

Before a competition, visualization will help you to be mentally prepared. By imagining yourself performing, your brain will adjust your heartbeat for the coming effort. Your hemoglobin level will increase, bringing more oxygen to your muscles and increasing your healing capacity. Your blood pressure will increase, and blood circulation will reach all your extremities, reducing accumulation of lactic acid. Endorphins will be released. This hormone has the power to decrease pain due to injury and gives a feeling of well-being along with a positive attitude. At this point, adrenaline is released and plays an important part in your whole metabolism; the resultant force, endurance, and speed will enhance your performance. If you can use all these assets before a competition, you will be more confident and will have a huge advantage over your opponent.

In competition, we can be in a defensive position or in an offensive position. Consider that reaction time is shorter than action time. Think of a Western movie where two cowboys are in a gunfight, one facing the other, ready to draw. Who has the greatest advantage, the one who draws first or the one who draws second? The time it takes to react is shorter than the time it takes to act. Therefore, the cowboy who draws his gun first is at a disadvantage.

Action calls for a voluntary command from the brain, while reaction calls on responses from the reflexes, which are not controlled by the brain. Instead, they are controlled by ganglions found at every nerve root extremity. These have the ability to imprint all repetitive movements and can instruct the muscles to execute a movement without going though the brain. Movements can therefore be executed at very high speed.

Imagine if all your movements, all your attack techniques, could be at reflex speed. During a competition, you can rarely assume a defensive position for very long. Sooner or later, you have to perform an offensive technique. By using feint techniques, your opponent's reaction time can be relatively slowed, giving you time to perform an action – an attack. But there is a way to perform a technique from an offensive position that can be as fast as a reaction technique. This becomes possible with visualization.

The time it takes to react is shorter than the time it takes to act.

A STATE OF ALERTNESS

As described above, our metabolism can be changed through visualization, as can our blood and hormone chemistry. I have also described how our state of mind can be modified to attain a level where we can perceive, feel, and unify our body and mind, as well as how sincerity can aid self-discovery, opening our hearts and minds to horizons never before explored, bringing us closer to enlightenment. Visualization can elevate our mind and body to an alert state in which the desired technique will be executed with a reflex-like speed, force, and precision.

Children use visualization without really knowing it. Their intellect is rarely solicited because they do not have a lot of life experience.

In contrast to an adult, who tries to reason through everything, the child's heart is closer to purity and wears practically no masks. Their expressions of emotion are spontaneous, and everything is expressed freely. They live in the present moment with intensity, having no fear of tomorrow, which for them is far away, just as their yesterday has long been forgotten.

Children are some of our best teachers in life. So many things can be learned from their behavior. Studying what makes an adult wear a mask, lack sincerity, and have difficulty dropping the mask, it seems worth putting energy into child development; so much can be won at that age. I say "won" because it often seems like we are losing the fight to remove our masks, which some of us have worn to help us get through certain stages in life that we find too hard to cross alone. These masks cannot be removed easily when they have been worn for many years. If we had known that, we would probably never have put them on.

Teaching visualization to young children enables them to realize at an early age that this exercise can be useful in understanding their inner emotions. They are then in a position to search for the origins of those emotions by preparing to face them without a mask. As they grow up, they are able to apply the visualization technique learned in taekwondo to their everyday lives.

At the end of each class I ask my students to sit on the floor, legs crossed, back straight, chin tucked in, and eyes closed. I tell them to see themselves executing the taekwondo technique they have just learned by adding as many details as possible. Sometimes I ask them to change their hair color in their imagination, or to imagine themselves with a blue mustache, and so on. The more often this is practiced, the more they start to connect with their soul, which in return brings self-confidence, calm, and love. When you have love in your heart, you get closer to nature, a step on the route toward enlightenment. You must stay in contact with that child who lives inside you. This is your true nature.

I don't believe that we should try to teach our own life philosophy to other people. Rather, we must teach them to find their own life philosophy, their own path. Visualization can be a marvelous tool to help us find our own philosophy since it helps us maintain contact with our soul.

Sincerity then becomes the first step we take. Without it, the image will be incomplete, and our eyes will not see what must be seen. To develop this state of mind, we must have a healthy body in which the mind and body become one, just like fire's light and heat. The mind and body must be in balance to lead us to enlightenment.

Success is in the attitude with which you choose to learn. Believing that you are perfect, that you have nothing left to learn, closes the door to knowledge. Visualization calls on the imagination. Visualization is the open door between mind and body. As the great scientist Albert Einstein said, "Imagination is more important than knowledge."

Imagination is more important than knowledge.

The *Do* of Taekwondo

Do signifies "the way" or "the path." It is what most distinguishes this art from other sports.

During its development over the last two thousand years, taekwondo has been greatly influenced by both war and peace. Because of this, taekwondo teaches both self-defense and harmony, which have great value for us today.

In the present day, psychological aggression is encountered more often than physical aggression. How many times have you been psychologically intimidated by a verbal attack, or suffered from stress? I'm sure this has happened to you often. Observe children's reactions in the schoolyard. There are always some children who are mistreated by others. These children become scapegoats even though they have done nothing wrong. The same thing happens when a person walks past a dog. If that person is scared, the dog will sense it. By observing a person's behavior, we can perceive whether he is vulnerable or not.

In taekwondo sparring, as a well-trained practitioner, you know how to cover your fear, or rather your insecurity, in front of your opponent. You know how to detect an opponent's lack of confidence and sense of security, and you will be able to direct his or her attack as you need to.

Our mental attitude is very important. But how can we acquire that confidence or sense of security that is so important? We must first develop mental balance and well-being within. In life, everything moves so fast that adaptation is extremely difficult. Then comes the insecurity phase, followed by a lack of self-confidence. We become vulnerable mentally as well as physically. How can we avoid this trap? We must take a journey inside ourselves and learn who we really are. We must discover our strengths to develop them; we must discover our weaknesses and learn how to make them our allies. To know ourselves, we must be sincere with ourselves and with others. We cannot act with our full potential as human beings if we do not act with sincerity. For the mind and body to be one, there must be sincerity. A practitioner who tries to perform for the wrong reasons (for example, to win praise) is not able to perform as well as if it were for a justified cause.

A lack of sincerity is an act against nature. It creates resistance within our bodies and consumes energy needlessly. We must be at peace with nature to live in balance. We must learn how to breathe, because breathing is the best way to communicate with nature. To understand this, we must know how to listen to nature and how to feel it. Only a sincere person will succeed at this. An incomparable serenity pervades you when this communication is established. You live an experience that makes you remember good childhood memories, moments in your life when life's daily headaches had not yet reached you. You will then be more aware of yourself. It is an ideal moment to reset your values, convictions, and objectives in life. In this way, taekwondo forces you to take an internal voyage. Many practitioners of this art realize it too late, and often quit before reaching this stage.

Taekwondo involves learning many physical techniques and requires a certain agility. When the student starts learning, the effort required is mainly physical. You need to work on your flexibility, coordination, endurance, distance, perception, and reflexes. This work often requires many years of effort. According to your development, this is how you, as a student, pass from the white belt to the yellow belt and climb the steps. As a general rule, when you have attained the red belt, you have reached a point where your physical skills are fully developed, meaning that your progress is at the stage where basically no change is noticeable. At first, you progress quickly, encouraged by seeing your efforts rewarded by the changing belt colors. But why does progress seem to cease at the red belt? It is often at that level that our physical development is at its maximum, and therefore progress is not very noticeable. This often makes students feel discouraged, and they quit, seeing no other issue at play.

The objective that most students aim for is to obtain their black belt. You start out full of determination, as everything is new and your progress is rapid due to the effort you make. But the higher you rise in the belt grading system, the more effort and discipline is required. If the only reward you seek is to obtain a black belt instead of being aware of the physical and psychological benefits that taekwondo provides, you will develop another problem. This happens to many students when they notice, after many years of work and effort, that their ambition was only greed. Feeling close to their goal, their effort decreases. They are content and satisfied with their position. A similar thing happens when a child wants to catch a ball rolling on the ground. Rushing to grab it and running toward it, when she gets close to it, her foot hits the ball and it rolls farther away. Some red-belt students, seeing themselves so close to that famous black belt they so covet, become satisfied with their position too soon and decrease the effort they had once made. By decreasing their effort, their progress declines, and they see things in disarray, their dream of being a black belt vanishing.

You must be aware and accept that physical effort alone is insufficient to obtain a black belt. The black belt symbolizes a certain balance, physically and mentally, that you must obtain. We become a black belt, we don't "have" a black belt. It represents evolution on the human plane. We become real, and we discover ourselves. Our self-perception becomes highly developed. We no longer see with the same eyes we used to see with. Our vision is now more elaborate, and we live fully.

We become a black belt, we don't "have" a black belt.

This is why you often hear about incredible feats by taekwondo masters even when they are of advanced age. They compensate for their lack of agility with the great wisdom they have developed.

You must make a transition so that your physical skills attain a certain level and your mind is trained to communicate more clearly with them. It is from this communication that you start to feel the balance that allows you to execute many movements with less energy. Your progress will then be greater than expected. You will feel in harmony and become further aware of the nature that surrounds you. Your taekwondo training will no longer have the same meaning, and your objectives will no longer be the same. What you feel inside is similar to what we feel when we fall in love. Everything surrounding us changes, and we feel good. Your state of mind is not the same as before; we call this state enlightenment. In this state, your intellect is at rest, and your real self, the subconscious, is wide awake. Training for the red belt is designed to allow you to attain this state of mind at will. A story follows to help you understand this.

THE NEW STUDENT

This tale is based on a classic Zen story, and takes place in the fourth century near a small village in Korea. At that time, taekwondo was only taught to a carefully selected few. The Dojang, the schools where taekwondo was taught, were part of monasteries.

For many years, a young boy had the ambition to become a taek-wondo student. Over the years he came regularly to the monastery doors where that art was being taught. When the master opened the door to him, the boy would always ask the same question: "Has the time come for me to be accepted as your student?"

"No, you are not ready," was the master's response.

As the boy got older, his desire to become a taekwondo student grew. One day he went to the monastery, as usual, anxious to ask the same question of the master. This time, the master answered in a severe tone, "Why do you want to be accepted?" Surprised by the question, the student was perplexed and hesitated to answer. Noticing the hesitation, the master said, "You are not ready; go away, and don't come back." As the master was closing the door, the student sincerely excused himself for disturbing the master and bowed before leaving. The master then opened the door and told him, "Now you are ready."

There is much to be learned from this story. Deep inside, the boy wanted to become a taekwondo student. He demonstrated ambition and perseverance. He had a goal and wanted to reach it. When the master asked him why, he was afraid to deceive the master and searched for the best possible answer. The student was full of desire, which often encourages greed and promotes a state of mind dominated by the intellect. The master expected an answer of sincerity, originating from his heart and not from his intellect. The master saw in the boy that his mind was in a state where his intellect was dominant. This state of mind does not allow the student to attain enlightenment. When the boy understood that he would never be admitted to the school, his dream vanished, eliminating his desire and making his intellect resign. At that moment, the boy's mind was in its purest state, in which he could perceive what his eyes could not show him before. His soul suddenly became sincere, and he was one with nature. The master knew how to recognize this state of mind.

When we are preoccupied, our intellect dominates. It is so centered on the problem at hand that it often sees no other issues, and therefore no solutions. When we take a long walk, the problem that had preoccupied us often vanishes, making room for the right solution. Movements done in a repetitive way become boring and tend to make our intellect resign. By resigning, our mind reaches a state that allows us to be more objective and to find our true nature. Taekwondo training is therefore oriented to allow you to reach that state of mind, to experience illumination, and to blossom. The student who masters that state possesses a mental power superior to that of others. This evokes another old Zen story:

THE MONK ON PILGRIMAGE

During the ninth century, two monks on pilgrimage were walking together along a river, observing nature. At that time, monks were strictly forbidden to talk to women. Near the river there was a beautiful young woman wearing a white silk dress. She wanted to cross the river but did not want her dress to get wet. One of the monks, in an attempt to help the woman, took her in his arms and crossed the river, leaving her on dry land on the other side. The monk crossed the river again to his friend, all the while maintaining his deep silence.

His friend was in shock. After several minutes of walking in silence, he said, "How could you disobey the rules? You have touched a woman. It's strictly prohibited."

The monk kept silent for a time, and then said, "I took that woman in my arms to help her safely reach dry land, and I deposited her on the opposite bank. You, my friend, are still carrying her."

This story is an example of mental power. The monk who carried the woman was capable of not allowing that act to disturb him. His act was legitimate, and the woman was in need. The act was natural, and the monk was therefore convinced of the legitimacy of his action. Once it was finished, his mind was ready to accomplish other tasks. His companion, on the other hand, was still haunted by the act, even though he had done nothing. He had lost control of his mind, and therefore demonstrated great weakness.

Without mental power, you are weak. There is no taekwondo without it. When I'm sparring, I can easily recognize the mental power of my opponents. Their eyes, their breathing, their shout

(Kihap), and their displacement are all ways we use to communicate, to spar. They are reflections of our minds.

People who are too confident in themselves are people with little mental power. An excess of self-confidence decreases the mind's perceptions. Here is a story to illustrate this fact.

THE LITTLE DUCK

A little duck hatched and saw daylight for the first time. His mother would regularly come to feed him. When he was strong enough, she brought him to swim with his older brothers and sisters. It was difficult at first because he had to overcome his fear of the unknown. He swam among his brothers and sisters, who protected and encouraged him.

During these outdoor activities, his mother kept an eye on him to ensure he was well. When she saw a stranger, she would group the family together to eliminate any potential danger. After a few days of outdoor activity, the little duck gained self-confidence, and on many occasions he led the family on the river. He enjoyed helping his mother keep the family safely together.

One day, a strange bird flew overhead. The little duck decided on his own to group his brothers and sisters together, even before his mother had made the decision. He wanted to impress her by showing her he could be in charge. His mother realized that it was time to put her child to the test. She brought him to a turbulent stream that she had already fully mastered. Because the stream was so rough, she had never taken her ducklings there to swim. But for this young duck, it was different. She felt that he needed this challenge to grow up.

He bounced with joy when he learned about the adventure his mother had planned for him. Arriving at the rapids, his heart started to beat hard and fast. The stream was very powerful. His mother described in great detail all the dangerous points of the river to prevent any injuries, and told him that she would wait for him downstream. Once his mother was gone, the little duck entered the water carefully. The first miles were difficult. Because of his determination, he was able to traverse the obstacles. He succeeded in perceiving the eddies to avoid them and to get around the rocks' sharp edges. A little bit further on the river got calmer. The little duck told himself that it was not as bad as he expected and started to play and fool around, while continuing to descend the river. Suddenly, he heard his mother's voice screaming at him to be careful. Right in front of him was a huge waterfall. He hurried to open his wings and flew to meet his mother in the air.

The little duck told his mother, "I thought that you were waiting for me downstream. How did you know I was in danger?"

"Well," she said, "when I described the dangerous parts of the river to you, I noticed that you were not paying full attention to my words. You were in too great a hurry to start and to show me that you are worthy to be the head of the family. You had too much self-confidence. So I decided to follow you in the sky. At first, you were paying attention to your surroundings. But later on, where the river got calmer, you got too self-confident, and that prevented you from noticing the danger ahead of you. Too much self-confidence changes our perception and judgment." After receiving this advice, the little duck understood the importance of mental power.

The *do* in taekwondo allows the development and possession of that mental power that helps us not only in sparring but also in everyday life. This *do* cannot simply be taught. You must feel it to discover your path and your philosophy. Your instructor is only a guide to help you on this journey toward your path. As a student you have a difficult task. You must discover yourself, develop your senses, and perceive. After you discover your soul, you will be able to discover the outside world. All this becomes an extremely rewarding experience.

I will end this chapter with a short classic story to help you with perception. It deals with being aware of the importance we attribute to certain emotions and how they can change our well-being.

THE VELVETEEN RABBIT

This is a story of a small boy who had a room full of toys of all kinds: electric trains, remote-controlled cars, electronic games, and so on. In this room there were also old toys: teddy bears, dolls, and an old wooden horse. After having amused his brothers and sisters, all these toys were put aside as they were worn out, slightly damaged, or just less attractive compared to the new motorized toys with colorful lights.

Among the toys was a velveteen rabbit. Missing an eye and with an arm slightly damaged and crumpled, the rabbit had known many hours of attention and care when the boy had been younger. He used to sleep with the child every night, always there to reassure him when he got scared during the night. When the boy was sad, he was there to listen and bring him comfort. He was always willing to play any game his best friend wanted to play. But now, for many months, the boy no longer noticed the rabbit, seeing only the shiny new electric toys.

One night, hearing the velveteen rabbit cry, the wooden horse asked him, "Why are you crying, little rabbit?"

The rabbit answered, "My friend doesn't love me anymore. He prefers the mechanical toys that make a lot of noise. He doesn't pick me up in his arms. I miss his love so much."

The wooden horse said, "Don't worry; you'll see. He did not forget you. I have known many children, as a matter of fact his brothers and sisters. They played with me for long hours. I have given them happiness and laughter. They loved me for many days and weeks, and now they have good memories. Even if they don't play with me anymore, I know that I have a special place in their hearts. It is what makes me real, and that is what matters most to me."

"What is real?" asked the rabbit.

"What is real," said the wooden horse, "is not that you are motorized or that you shine like all those new toys. Those toys are artificial. They are hard, have sharp edges, and break easily. To be real is that it does not bother you to be slightly damaged, to have a missing eye or even a torn shoulder. You are damaged because you have been caressed by the love a child had toward you. To be real is for the one who loves you always to find you beautiful. His eyes see that you are damaged, but his heart feels even more love for you. To be real is to have a place in someone's heart."

The little rabbit was comforted by this. Every day he would remember the nice moments he had known being with the boy.

He would always have a special place in his heart for him. He could accept that the child would come into the room to get other toys to play with. He told himself that even though those toys were in the boy's hands, he was in the boy's heart.

A day came when the child did not come to get toys from the room. The rabbit started to worry about his dear friend. The next morning, the rabbit heard someone knocking at the door of the house. It was the doctor who had come to see the boy. The rabbit overheard the doctor tell the boy's mother that he was very sick and had a high fever. "The boy must stay in bed until his fever drops," he said. The boy was scared to stay alone in his room, and his mother could not be there all the time. She went into the playroom to search for a teddy bear to keep the boy company. She noticed the little velveteen rabbit. She did not really know why, but she felt something special in the little rabbit. She took it with her.

The little rabbit trembled with joy when he was in the boy's room once again. A tear fell from the rabbit's eye. The boy was trembling with fever and was sweating so much that his pajamas were wet. But this did not matter to the rabbit. He just wanted to be as close as possible to his beloved friend.

The boy's mother said, "Look, I brought you the little velveteen rabbit that you used to sleep with when you were little." A big smile came to the boy's face, and his eyes sparkled with joy. He took the rabbit and held it close to his heart. He remembered all the nice times he had had with the velveteen rabbit. All these forgotten memories came back to life. The rabbit vibrated with joy. He understood what the wooden horse had tried to explain to him. He felt warmth come over him because he had a place in the boy's heart.

During the night, the rabbit could not fall asleep because the boy was too restless. Sometimes he was warm, sometimes he was cold. Even with all his discomfort, the boy did not let go of the rabbit. He held him tightly to his heart. This went on for three days. Even though he could not fall asleep, the rabbit had never felt so happy. He was very dedicated to his role, the help he was bringing the boy. Deep communication existed even if no words were spoken.

On the fourth day, the boy's fever broke. He started to play with the little rabbit. He showed him some affection. The boy knew that during his days of illness, the little rabbit had stayed close to him. The new toys did not interest him anymore.

The doctor came to see the boy. "He is better, and tomorrow he will be allowed to play outside," said the doctor. Leaving the boy's room, the doctor told his mother, "Everything that was in contact with the boy during his sickness must be burned to destroy the germs."

During this last night, the rabbit slept near the heart of the one he loved, to whom he had given himself without reservation.

The following morning, when the boy came down to the kitchen for breakfast, the gardener went up to his room, at the mother's request, to take out everything that had come into contact with the boy during his illness. The rabbit, along with many other objects, was put in a wheelbarrow to be burned. The rabbit was very sad. He knew he would never see his dear friend again. But remembering what the wooden horse had told him, he started to think of the good memories he had of his last days near his friend. Even if he was going to die, he knew that he would live on in the boy's heart.

Suddenly, the gardener hit a rock with the wheelbarrow, and the velveteen rabbit fell out. The gardener did not notice and continued on his way to burn the wheelbarrow's contents. The velveteen rabbit had fallen near a tree. After breakfast, the boy went to his room to play with his rabbit. To his surprise, his bedding and blankets were gone. Even the curtains were missing. Not finding his rabbit, he called to his mother. She explained why she had had to burn everything, including the velveteen rabbit.

Crying, the boy fell to the floor, devastated, yelling, "I want my rabbit back!" He did not want to play anymore. Even though his mother brought him his bright new toys, he showed no interest in them.

The velveteen rabbit could not move from where he had fallen, but he filled his thoughts with the love he felt for the boy. Suddenly two rabbits bounced out of the forest. Seeing the velveteen rabbit, they started to laugh. "Look at that rabbit. He doesn't even have feet," said one of them. "It is a velveteen rabbit, a toy. He's not real," replied the other. At this, they left the velveteen rabbit in his distress.

For many days, the boy did nothing other than to think of his velveteen rabbit. The place the rabbit held in his heart grew so much that the rabbit started to feel something very extraordinary. His feet started to grow. It was true, he was growing real feet! His eye and his arms started to be mobile. He was becoming real.

All the emotions that linked the velveteen rabbit and the boy grew to such a level that one could question what reality was. The velveteen rabbit could now jump around like a real rabbit. He went back to the boy's house. When the boy saw him, he recognized him right away. He took him in his arms and caressed him. The rabbit felt the boy's heart beating, and for the first time the boy felt the rabbit's living heartbeat. With much care he put the rabbit on the ground, accepting that his place now was in the forest. The rabbit looked the boy in his eyes, understood, and left.

Both knew that they would always be united in their hearts. With this experience, the boy grew up. He did not only look with his eyes but with his heart. In this way he could discover himself and discover the world around him.

Mental Conditioning

Do we want a huge reserve of energy? Are we searching to accomplish great feats to outdo ourselves? Excellent physical conditioning is required, and it is the first step of our training. But what about conditioning the mind?

Physical conditioning has its limits, which is why we must complement our physical training program with mental training or "mental conditioning." How can we discipline our minds? We must start by having a disciplined lifestyle. If you work in a methodical way and put everything in order, your mind becomes trained with a certain discipline. If you get used to walking with the right posture, sit straight, and so on, you allow your lungs to function properly, which will help you get good blood oxygenation, essential for brain function. It will also prevent future back pain. As I explain in the chapter on the digestive system, in addition to oxygen, essential elements are required for the brain.

After reaching the best possible brain efficiency through proper nutrition and oxygenation, we are ready to train the mind. We need exercises that demand a lot of mental energy; taekwondo classes are oriented toward this kind of exercise. That is why many young students of taekwondo notice a distinct improvement in their concentration and consequently their school results. For adults, work efficiency should improve for the same reason. When the body is disciplined, the mind also becomes disciplined. We must make it work and require the mind to accomplish extremely difficult tasks to develop harmony with the body. The mind and the body must be as one.

It is like the flame of a fire, which unifies two different energy sources: heat and light. Nevertheless, the fire becomes only one source of energy when both are united. Similarly, human beings can unify two different sources of energy: mental and physical. If a union in perfect harmony does not exist, there will be imbalance, and the individual will not be able to experience enlightenment, which we all deserve in this life.

Mental conditioning permits the mind to communicate with the entire body. Before a confrontation, whether it is in sports or not, we need certain mental conditioning. If I must spar with an opponent, I must reunite all my energies. I must visualize the match, imagining myself in action. I must feel with my whole body the techniques that I will deliver before their real execution. This will get my body prepared, and the communication between my mind and body will open and allow the information through.

This principle applies to everyday circumstances as well. Whether I am making a presentation at a conference or executing a taekwondo technique, I need mental conditioning. Before strenuous exercise, we warm up our muscles for better performance. But it is important not to forget the mental conditioning, which is equally important. It is simple: we only need to visualize ourselves in action. Further details are provided in the "Visualization" chapter.

Kihap: Why Shout?

Animals use various loud sounds to demonstrate their superiority over an opponent. Often no physical contact happens after an animal makes its particular sound; lions roar and dogs bark to bring an opponent's attention to their mental power and determination.

One of the first things that spectators notice about taekwondo is the shout when we are sparring. This shout is called **Kihap,** and it differs from the shouts or yells used in other martial arts because of its specific objective: to concentrate energy on one single point and to release it as quickly as possible while allowing all the body's tension to release once the technique is completed. This is done to allow a combination with another technique or to displace the body in such a way that the center of gravity will not be lowered.

The shout allows us to unify our physical and mental energy. To shout is natural. If you frighten a child or even an adult, in response they will shout. The act of shouting engages a chemical reaction in each of us. Even animals, when faced with a stressful situation, will shout (or roar, bark, or cry) before and after a battle. Observe a taekwondo class. Just by listening to the students' Kihap, you will be able to distinguish the beginners from the advanced. The

Kihap reflects the mind's power. If it is timid, the technique will lack conviction.

The shout also has a psychological effect on your opponent. A well-performed Kihap reveals your mental power to your opponent when you're sparring. This can have the effect of breaking your opponent's concentration. This is also why the Kihap is done before as well during the attack. The shout is important because it brings a feeling of confidence and also releases your tension before an attack.

One of the most important actions provided by the Kihap is the chemical reaction inside you. Executed with the unification of your mind and body, the Kihap stimulates your body in a specific way. When your concentration is at its maximum and you are in a combat situation, all body systems that are not necessary at that moment are temporarily suspended; the stomach sphincter closes, and digestion and intestinal activities stop. The reason for this is to reduce all unnecessary energy use so that energy is focused on the muscles, which must be able to supply their maximum capacity. Energy is produced using **oxygen** and **sugar** in a kind of combustion. The lungs dilate to increase oxygen and carbon dioxide exchange; the liver releases sugar in the form of glycogen that it has stored in reserve; and the blood pressure increases due to the contraction of blood vessels, permitting blood to flow to the farthest muscle cells in the legs, arms, and back. The heart rate increases up to 150 beats per minute and on some occasions can reach 200 beats per minute. The brain receives increased blood flow for better reflexes and especially to react faster. The blood increases its clotting ability to minimize bleeding in case of injury. Obviously, all this happens when your concentration level and mental conditioning are at their peak and ready for action.

The Kihap was not only developed and used in taekwondo. Look at animals in combat; all the **chemistry** described above is happening in them. They have a natural sound to make that reflects their mental power. This is their instinct for survival.

The Kihap brings me well-being in my training. It frees my accumulated tensions after a hard day of work. I feel my mind and body unify. My mind becomes relaxed after such training; I feel part of nature, and I feel alive.

Without Kihap, energy can't be delivered at its maximum.

This is why Kihap is so important in taekwondo. Without Kihap, energy can't be delivered at its maximum. How is Kihap performed? We must learn how to breathe. We start with breathing exercises. To facilitate them, I will divide the breathing region in two sections:

1. The thoracic cage

2. The abdomen

Under normal conditions, we should breathe with the abdominal region, the lower belly. To feel this technique, sit down on the floor, legs crossed and back straight. Place your left hand on your abdomen, slightly above the navel. Your right hand is placed on your thoracic cage, between the nipples. Now breathe normally. Only your left hand should rise, and your right hand should practically remain immobile. Repeat this breathing exercise until it becomes natural. You'll soon notice that this kind of breathing gives you a feeling of relaxation and will help you rest. It is a practical technique to help people fall asleep. A crying baby will often be relieved when you gently apply pressure to the abdomen with your hand. The baby then needs to push slightly with the abdomen to restore breathing to its natural way.

Several glands can be stimulated by such breathing, which helps explain its benefits. Look at a person who is frightened or even hysterical. Pay attention to the breathing. It becomes rapid and short and originates mainly from the thoracic cage with little abdominal movement. Such breathing prevents adequate carbon dioxide and oxygen exchange. This is called hyperventilation and can lead to a loss of consciousness. In this case, we have to help the person find normal abdominal breathing.

When you have mastered this first breathing technique, you will be ready for the second technique, which I call forced abdominal breathing.

FORCED ABDOMINAL BREATHING

This kind of breathing is not natural and must be seen as an exercise. It has several objectives that make it useful in helping us maintain good health and developing our concentration level.

First, sit on the floor or on a chair. As you master this technique, you should be able to practice it standing up or lying down, even without the use of your hands. Place your left hand on your abdomen, slightly above the navel. Your right hand is placed on your thoracic cage, between the nipples. When breathing in, contract your abdominal muscles in such a way as to bring your belly inside, without inflating the thoracic cage. In other words, as you inhale you should feel your abdomen going in, with the help of your left hand. During that time your right hand, which is over your thoracic cage, should stay immobile, since you should not be using these muscles to take in air. As you exhale, you should force the abdomen out, carefully minimizing the movement of the thoracic cage. Your hands will allow you to feel the abdominal and thoracic movement.

This exercise is relatively difficult to master. It helps us to be conscious of abdominal breathing, which has an important physiological role. The technique permits massage of our abdominal organs, including the liver, pancreas, stomach, and intestines, promoting organ cleansing. You can practice this exercise periodically during the day, and you should soon feel its benefits.

Reflexology

Reflexology is a therapeutic massage technique that focuses on certain reflex points, permitting energy to circulate liberally, improving circulation, promoting relaxation, and allowing a decrease or even elimination of pain.

In this science, we learn that the feet contain reflex points. They are in reality small nerve endings that the different organs of our body use to eliminate their toxins through the lymphatic system. Our body is built this way because human beings evolved to walk barefoot. Consequently, walking barefoot on rough surfaces massaged these reflex points continually and naturally. When an organ does not function normally, it accumulates a type of crystal on the nerve endings. This massage technique works to break down the crystals into very small particles that can be eliminated by the lymphatic system.

As a reflexologist certified by the Reflexology Association of Canada, I have practiced this form of natural medicine since 1989. Reflexology is a complex science that originated in Asia. My intent is not to go into too much detail since that could easily fill an entire book. I do want to point out certain techniques that may help you.

We consider the arch of the foot to act like a second heart. This means that when you walk, certain muscles in the arch are put to work and help the blood flow up the legs to the heart. This blood then flows through blood vessels in the lungs to exchange carbon dioxide for oxygen. Foot muscles often become tense, and foot massage is recommended to treat the reflex points and relax the muscles. A reflexology session must always start with massage techniques because to reach the deep reflex points, the muscles must be relaxed.

There are reflex points in different parts of the body, but we will discuss only the ones found in the feet since they have negative energy levels; this means that the best results are obtained at the feet. Foot massage will increase blood circulation, which is necessary for any athlete. Relaxation, of course, is another benefit.

When you receive a massage, you must be sitting or lying on your back. First contact must be made with your left foot, which is more receptive for a relaxation massage; for a deep massage of the reflex points, the right foot is most receptive. Before starting the massage, it is important to remove all metallic objects that are in contact with the skin, including jewelry, money, watches, and keys, because metal can interfere with the transmission of energy. Some lotion or oil can be used to make the massage more enjoyable.

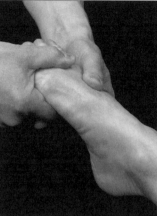

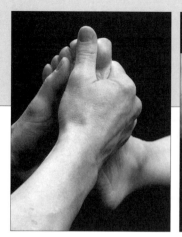

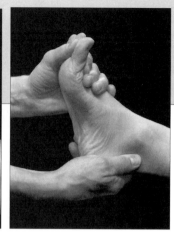

EFFLEURAGE

The first technique is called effleurage. The foot is pulled toward the masseur during the massage, and both hands must be in contact with the foot. Effleurage is performed as if applying lotion to the foot and rubbing it in. Hand movements must be slow and delicate.

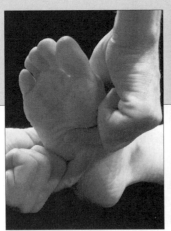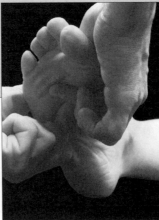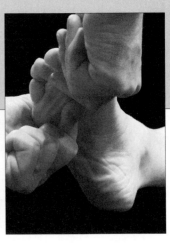

SWEEPING

The second technique is sweeping, which is performed under the foot as well as on top of the foot, slightly pulled toward the masseur. To sweep the bottom of the foot, both palms are placed on top of the foot with the index fingers under the foot. With the help of both index fingers, a kind of rotation is performed, one index finger after the other, overlapping, from the heel to the toes.

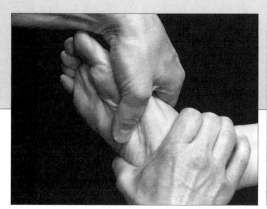 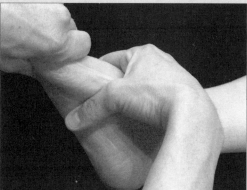

LATERAL TORSION

The third technique is lateral torsion, similar to wringing water out
of a cloth by twisting it with both hands. Both hands are placed
side by side on the inside of the foot, with both thumbs under
the foot and the other fingers on top. Motion is a few repetitions
from the heel toward the toes and from the toes toward the heel
of a light twisting movement so that pressure from the right hand
is felt toward the top and pressure from the left hand is toward
the bottom. During the twisting, the masseur applies light pressure
that tends to separate the hands. This technique slightly pulls the
foot and relieves much tension.

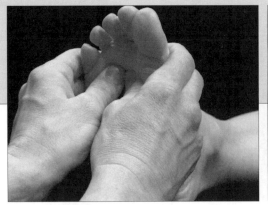
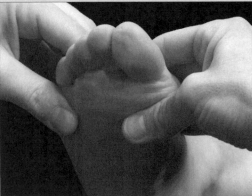

THE BUTTERFLY

The fourth technique is the butterfly, in which both thumbs, one in front of the other, are placed under the foot, and the fingers on top. Continuously pulling the foot toward him – or herself, the masseur makes a closing movement with the fingers followed by a closing movement with the thumbs. This butterfly movement is done slowly. The opening movement is done while the receiver and the masseur breathe in; the closing is done while they exhale. The action is repeated a few times.

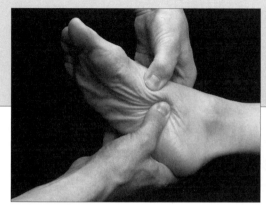 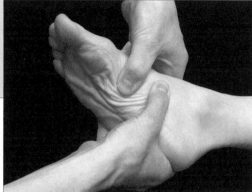

THE CROSSED CATERPILLAR

The fifth technique is the crossed caterpillar. This massage technique is practiced along the inside of the arch, beginning at the big toe and moving toward the heel. The foot is held with both hands with the fingers on either side, except the thumbs, which cross each other. The thumbs rejoin each other on the arch in a movement similar to two caterpillars crawling, until they cross and pass each other. The massage technique is repeated from the base of the big toe down to the heel.

Afterward, the movement is started again, this time with only small circular movements of the thumb moving along the arch.

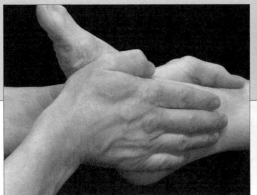
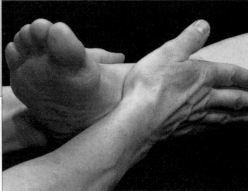

MALLEOLI

The sixth technique involves the malleoli, which are the protruding bones on either side of the ankle. Both palms are placed on the bones. The masseur gently pulls and maintains the pulling pressure with the inside part of the hands. The massage starts slowly with the right hand rising while the left hand descends, then vice versa.

The foot will move from left to right, and the technique is repeated for approximately 12 seconds.

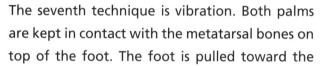

VIBRATION

The seventh technique is vibration. Both palms are kept in contact with the metatarsal bones on top of the foot. The foot is pulled toward the masseur, who creates a back-and-forth movement that makes the foot gently vibrate. This movement must be done while exhaling. Repeat three times.

Once these techniques are completed for both feet, always starting with the left foot – which is more receptive to first contact – a small effleurage massage is done on the right foot – which is more receptive to deeper massages and reflex points – gently pulled toward the masseur.

After that, we are ready to examine the condition of the reflex points. Each reflex point represents an organ or gland in the body. My objective is not to train reflexologists, but I would like to present the techniques, which are easily adaptable if you want to perform them on yourself or a friend. These techniques can aid in your well-being through relaxing massage or the treatment of congested reflex points.

As a reflexologist, I intervene to stimulate or calm certain organs or glands to allow healing or relief for my patients. To achieve this, specific deep knowledge of human anatomy and pathology is required. What I want to teach is simply to intervene in a neutral way to allow the reflex points to operate normally. the following picture outlines the reflex points of diffe-rent organs and glands in the body.

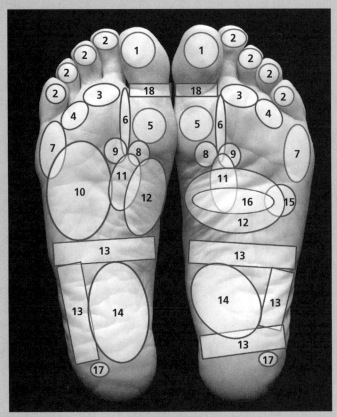

Principal reflex-point zones on the bottom of the foot

1 Head

2 Sinuses

3 Eyes

4 Ears

5 Heart

6 Esophagus and lungs

7 Shoulders

8 Adrenal glands

9 Solar plexus

10 Liver

11 Kidneys

12 Stomach

13 Colon

14 Intestines

15 Spleen

16 Pancreas

17 Sciatic nerve

18 Neck

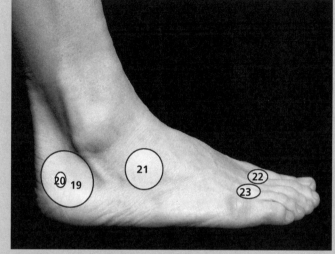

Principal reflex-point zones on the outside of the foot

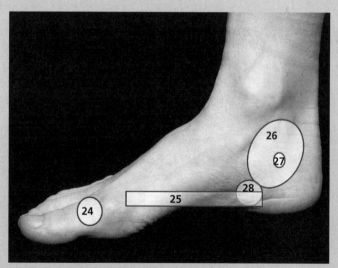

Principal reflex-point zones on the inside of the foot

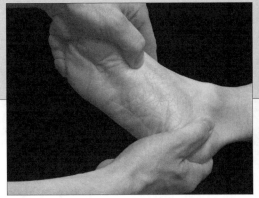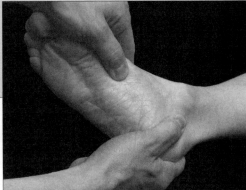

THE CATERPILLAR WALK

The first technique used to reveal congested reflex points is the caterpillar walk. We always start on the right foot, which is more receptive to deep massage. Remember that a relaxation massage must be done prior to starting. Ideally a session starts with a relaxation massage of the left foot. The recipient is kept covered so that the feet do not get cold. The right foot is massaged to relax, and then a deep massage can start.

The foot is gently pulled toward the masseur with both hands. The thumb makes a caterpillar-walk movement under, over, and on the side of the foot, seeking any painful points. The recipient informs the practitioner of any pain felt, identifying the pain level on a scale of 1 to 10.

Note that treating more than three reflex points per foot is not recommended, and a reflexology treatment session should not be done more than twice per week. The reason is that the objective of massaging the reflex points is to break down toxic crystals into very small particles. These fine particles will travel though the lymphatic system to be eliminated, which takes a certain amount of time. Not exceeding two sessions that treat three reflex points per foot allows a reasonable time for the lymphatic system to accomplish the task. This elimination time is not required for relaxation massages, which can be performed more frequently.

Now back to the reflex-point massage. By this point the recipient should have noted the painful points on a scale of 1 to 10. Choose the three most painful points to massage. Always start with the one closest to the toes and work toward the heel. Once you have located a point according to the pain felt by the recipient, you are ready to break down the toxins into small particles. To achieve this, press firmly on the reflex point with your thumb, executing a movement in the form of a horizontal figure 8 (∞). Your thumb must not slide on the skin, so the skin follows your movement. This technique is practiced while the foot is continuously gently pulled toward the masseur.

The recipient breathes out slowly, and at the same time concentrates on the pain felt and diffuses it mentally on a large surface in order to decrease it. The technique is applied three times during three exhalations, taking care to release the pressure of the thumb as the recipient inhales. The masseur must also synchronize breathing out with the recipient. To achieve this, watch the abdomen. Inhale when you see the recipient's abdomen rise. Breathe out when the recipient does, and at the same time, apply pressure with the thumb in the horizontal-figure-8 movement covering the reflex point without sliding on the skin. When the recipient breathes in, the abdomen inflates; release the pressure on the reflex point and breathe in. Repeat this three times for each reflex point.

After massaging each reflex point, you must do a little relaxation massage using the effleurage and sweeping techniques. These provide immense relief from the pain caused by the reflex-point massage.

The position of your hands during the reflex-point massage is very important. The hands should touch each other while applying pressure, and usually they touch each other at the fingers. Contact with just one finger is sufficient. The reason is to close your energy loop, so that your negative energy will not be given to the recipient, and the recipient's negative energy will not affect you.

Once the reflex-point massage is completed, start over on the relaxation massage using the techniques previously described, under the foot as well as on top of it.

CALF MASSAGE

Extend the massage to the calf using the caterpillar-walk technique with effleurage on each side of the calf, starting from the heel.

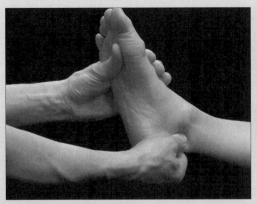
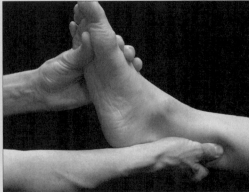

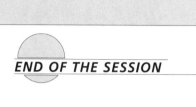

END OF THE SESSION

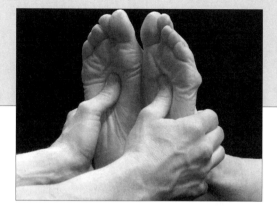

Once the massage of the right foot is completed, the same process is repeated on the left foot, after covering the right foot in order to keep it warm. Start again with a light relaxation massage before searching for the reflex points that need to be treated.

When both feet and calves have been massaged, you are ready to end the session. To do so, it is important to help the patient reach a level of relaxation. Hold the right foot with the left hand, and the left foot with the right hand. The thumb of each hand is placed under the feet, slightly above the center. Place yourself so that your arms are bent at a 90-degree angle.

Each time the recipient breathes out, by moving your upper body you apply pressure with the thumbs for the length of the entire exhalation. Breathe out at the same time the recipient does. Release the pressure when you inhale. This technique must be repeated ten times. It is very calming, and it is useful when people have anxiety.

In this chapter, I have tried to simplify certain reflexology techniques to help you benefit from the well-being this science can provide. Like many exercises, these techniques require practice. You will find the results are surprising.

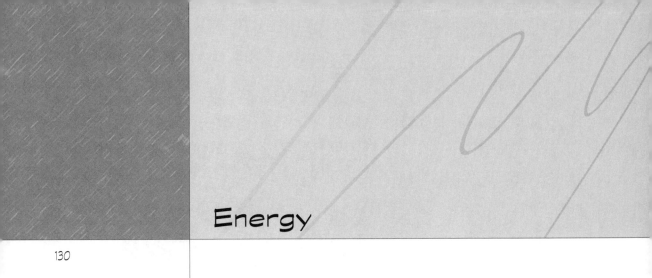

Energy

The body needs energy to function. This energy is largely supplied through the nutrients we consume.

MUSCULAR COMBUSTION

The nutrients in food are divided into three categories:

1. PROTEINS

These supply no immediately available energy except, in a very limited way, in exercise that requires great strength. They build the essential components of our tissues. The body has no way to store them in reserve.

2. LIPIDS (FATS)

A secondary energy source, particularly for tasks requiring endurance, lipids are accumulated in the muscles, under the skin, and around the internal organs.

3. CARBOHYDRATES (SUGARS)

Carbs are an essential combustible during exercise. The body accumulates them in the form of glycogen in the muscles and in the liver. When effort is exerted, muscles cannot sufficiently absorb energy nutrients to replace what they burn. This is why athletes have greater endurance during competition when they have greater reserves of accumulated glycogen in the body. Training is thus oriented to the principle that the more frequently muscles burn their glycogen reserves, the more their reserves will increase. The greater the glycogen stores, the more able the athlete is to apply sustained effort.

But muscles can only store a limited amount of glycogen. Can we continue to improve our endurance after this limit has been reached? What is interesting here is that when the muscles frequently burn their glycogen reserves, they become used to it, and with time they start to burn more fat during exertion. This economizes on the glycogen reserves. The combustion of fat combined with the glycogen stored in the muscles provides a result superior to glycogen consumption alone. This is why repetitive training allows a decrease of fat in the body. Otherwise the body cannot burn fat and can only use glycogen and blood sugar as a source of energy.

This explains why a person with a poor aerobic system has difficulty losing weight. They need to train in a way that increases their aerobic endurance. At that point, when doing endurance exercises, the system better burns fat as a source of energy.

I often use the term **burn**. When we want to burn a piece of wood, one of the essential elements involved is oxygen. No combustion is possible without oxygen. The term *burn* here implies **consumption**. But consumption is only achieved with a sufficient oxygen supply, which allows a specific chemical reaction and the transformation of a substance into energy.

The muscles burn fat and glycogen, transforming them into energy. They need oxygen to do this. Oxygen is transported to the muscles with the help of the red blood cells (hemoglobin) that nourish them. This is why, to increase our energy capacity, it is necessary to have a cardiovascular system that is in shape. Our exercise program must promote the burning of the glycogen reserves in our muscles. To achieve this we must:

Strengthen the cardiac muscles to increase blood flow
Enlarge the arterioles to allow blood to circulate in larger quantities
Increase the number and size of red blood cells to carry more oxygen
Increase the rate of oxygen absorption from the blood into the muscles through enzymes in the muscles

Lactic Acid

When it burns, glycogen forms a product called pyruvic acid. If exercise is performed at an intensity where the oxygen supply is sufficient, pyruvic acid is transformed into carbon dioxide to be eliminated by the respiratory system and partially by the kidneys (in the form of urine). This is called the **aerobic** system.

On the other hand, if exercise is so intense or accelerated in a way that the oxygen supply becomes deficient, pyruvic acid is transformed into lactic acid, which accumulates in the muscles and then crosses into the blood. This acid is detrimental to muscular contraction to the point that it becomes more and more difficult for the muscles to function. The athlete will feel fatigue, and eventually pain increases dramatically to the point that muscle cramps may develop. This is called **anaerobic** exercise.

One piece of advice I give my students to prevent this anaerobic condition is to pay attention to their breathing. If their breathing becomes rapid and they start to gasp during an exercise, it means the body is lacking oxygen. It is better to decrease the rate or intensity of the exercise. In aerobic exercise, you should be able to talk relatively freely during the exertion.

After intense training, we must always perform a little aerobic exercise to allow the blood to circulate more easily to every extremity in the body. In this way, a good proportion of the lactic acid can be eliminated without having too badly damaged the muscles.

Digestion

We know that nutrients in food are divided in three categories:

- **PROTEINS**
- **FATS**
- **CARBOHYDRATES**

To understand how nutrition works, we have to know about the fundamental principles of our digestive system. If we don't have proper nutrition, even the best training program won't allow us to attain our full energy potential. Briefly, this is how digestion occurs.

Inside the body is a chemical laboratory that is among the most complex in the world. It is the digestive system, which comprises extraordinary organs that, after a series of chemical reactions and mechanical work, transform the nutrients in food into simple soluble substances to allow them to nourish the cells of the body. As athletes we want our food to supply the necessary energy to perform and repair the tissues damaged through sports. We must select our food with great care; digesting it can consume our energy instead of supplying us with more.

THE MOUTH

THE TEETH

- **Incisors:** used to cut (8)

- **Canines:** used to tear (8)

- **Premolars:** act like a jackhammer (4)

- **Molars:** used to chew (12)

THE TONGUE

The tongue is equipped with a strong muscle that serves to mix food with saliva. With the help of little protuberances called papilla, we have the sense of taste and are able to sense temperature and texture.

TASTE

There are four tastes:

- **Sweet:** sensed on the tip of the tongue

- **Acid:** sensed on the sides of the tongue

- **Bitter:** sensed on the back of the tongue

- **Salty:** sensed all over the tongue

CHEWING

Chewing is needed to grind the food with the teeth and to stir it with the tongue. The salivary glands excrete enzymes to produce a mix for later digestion.

SALIVA

The purpose of saliva is primarily to liquefy food. Amylase and ptyalin (enzymes found in saliva) partially digest starch. Up to

50 percent of starch can be digested if food is chewed properly. This is why it is preferable not to drink at the same time as eating, because saliva is diluted and starch will be less digested.

To increase saliva secretion, meal presentation is important. We must look at what we are eating and take time to smell it. This excites our senses and activates our salivary glands. We must eat in a calm atmosphere.

Many children swallow pasta (and other food) whole without even chewing it. Pasta contains mainly starch, and if it isn't chewed, it remains practically undigested, because starch is largely digested in the mouth with the help of saliva. What we swallow should be mostly in liquid form.

THE PHARYNX

The pharynx is where air and food meet. It is important to chew our food properly, to mix it adequately with saliva, and to swallow it calmly, with the back straight, to prevent it taking the wrong path.

THE ESOPHAGUS

The esophagus is a tube composed of muscular fibers that contract, or perform peristalsis, to help food descend toward the stomach. The esophagus comes in contact with the spinal column and follows its curves. If you don't pay attention to your posture, you may have difficulty in digestion.

THE STOMACH

The largest organ of the body, the stomach has strong musculature to provide grinding functions. The stomach is situated in the lower left part of the abdominal cavity under the diaphragm. It looks like a pleated bag approximately ten inches deep in the shape of a J. The stomach has unique stretching capacity.

The stomach permits gastric secretions of hydrochloric acid to mix with food. It is in the stomach that the protein starts to digest. Sugars are digested largely in the small intestine. This is why it is preferable not to consume meals rich in sugars or glucose and rich in protein at the same time. I will clarify that subject in the section on "Nutritional Combinations."

THE SMALL INTESTINE

Twenty-three to twenty-six feet in length and one inch wide, the small intestine has approximately fifteen to twenty intestinal loops. It is situated in the central abdominal cavity and ends on the right side with the very important ileocecal valve. It is divided into three sections:

1. **The duodenum:** where bile and pancreatic secretions are released. The duodenum is approximately eight to fifteen inches in length.

2. **The jejunum:** approximately eight to ten feet in length

3. **The ileum:** approximately eleven feet in length

The jejunum and ileum are characterized by mucous and include multitudes of small fibrous pleats called intestinal villi, which are similar to hairs and have the appearance of velvet. Various gastric juices are secreted here and transform the food, assisted by the small glands at the ends of the villi so that its nutrients can be transported by capillaries to larger blood vessels. Only vitamins and minerals take this route. As soon as fats arrive in the capillaries, they are moved by the lymphatic network, which circulates slowly throughout the body. Sugars and proteins, once broken down by different secretions, are transported to the liver by a large blood vessel called the hepatic portal vein.

THE LARGE INTESTINE

Measuring approximately five feet in length, it is divided into four sections:

1. Right ascending colon

2. Horizontal transverse colon

3. Left descending colon

4. Rectum, terminated by the anus

The colon contains no enzymes; rather it contains bacteria. Its principle role is the recovery of the water used for digestion and the accumulation of fecal matter for evacuation (bowel movement).

The bacteria in the colon, called intestinal flora, combat rotting food and increase immunity against many types of disease. This explains why people who consume large amounts of sugar – which tends to disrupt our intestinal flora – may be more susceptible to infections. Antibiotics and chemicals alter the colon's environment considerably. Intestinal flora may also be very sensitive to our emotions.

Food eaten in excess causes certain nutrients to be insufficiently transformed in the large intestine, allowing it to rot, especially if the food contains low fiber. Yogurt, fiber, and fermentation products help maintain normal and healthy intestinal flora. It can also help rebuild the flora. As a phytotherapist, I often recommend plain yogurt when people suffer from infections or when they are taking antibiotics. Considering that intestinal flora is sensitive to our emotions, consuming yogurt and decreasing our intake of refined foods, which are rich in sugar, can decrease our risk of infection during stressful periods or when we are traveling.

Have I been able to make you aware of all the hard work your body needs to accomplish just for digestion? While digestion is going on, we want to have sufficient energy to accomplish our daily activities. As an athlete, if you dream of attaining your maximum energy level, you have to take the time to consider the energy that is spent on digestion. A small amount of work invested in proper nutrition will pay off in energy gain. This includes eating foods rich in vitamins and minerals.

In summary, the least-refined foods are the most nutritious and provide the most energy. The body must be able to digest food with little effort and energy. Taekwondo is a discipline on the physical and mental plane. Consequently the black-belt holder is not only a balanced person but is also physically and psychologically disciplined. This discipline is equally reflected in our lifestyles and nutritional styles. We must conform to nature's laws; when we are hungry, we eat wisely, in a healthy way, and with reasonable, well-balanced portions.

Proper Nutrition

Certain nutrients are essential for the proper functioning of the body:

1. **Carbohydrates and forms of sugar**

2. **Lipids and fatty acids**

3. **Proteins and amino acids**

4. **Water**

5. **Vitamins**

6. **Minerals and trace elements**

Energy and heat sources:	**Catalysts and regulators:**
• Carbohydrates (starches and sugars)	• Vitamins
• Lipids (fats)	• Dietary minerals
	• Fiber
	• Water

Construction and supporting materials:
• Proteins
• Dietary minerals
• Water

CARBOHYDRATES

Carbohydrates and sugars are absorbed in the small intestine in the form of simple sugars or glucose. Disaccharides and complex sugars must be transformed by digestion. This may take up to thirty minutes to occur.

SIMPLE SUGARS

Fruits, vegetables, and honey are a few examples of sources of simple sugars called glucose and fructose.

Milk is another source of simple sugar called galactose.

Important: Simple concentrated sugars should be avoided because they are absorbed rapidly. They disrupt the glucose level in the blood and add stress to the liver and pancreas. This stress creates an overload of work for these organs to establish normal blood sugar levels.

DISACCHARIDES ("DOUBLE SUGARS")

Syrups and molasses are examples of double sugars, called sucrose or saccharose.

Milk also contains a double sugar called lactose.

Malt syrup is another example of a double sugar called maltose.

An example : you eat an apple. From what was previously described, we know how it is digested. As this is occurring, the thyroid gland acts as a conductor for your body. The thyroid receives information on whether your blood sugar level is normal. As the sugar level increases, it intervenes to prevent an excess of blood sugar. For an apple, the thyroid orders the pancreas to secrete a small amount of insulin, which allows a small amount of sugar to be stored in the cells and maintain blood sugar at a normal level. Your body does not notice this occurring. The apple is rich in sugar in the form of fructose (fruit sugar) and minerals. The apple is an excellent source of energy. It has the advantage of having nutritional fiber, which slows down its assimilation. Fiber also gives volume to your stool, which helps with evacuating the intestines. Up to this point, everything seems to be working well, and you feel good and energetic.

This time, think of drinking a glass of apple juice instead of eating an apple. Things can go somewhat wrong here. The juice of ten apples may be necessary to fill a glass, which changes the scenario. The thyroid analyzes the situation as in the previous case, but since the glass of juice contains less fiber than the apples that contained it, the body assimilates the juice faster. Imagine how you would feel if you had eaten ten apples one after the other. You would have felt satisfied for a much longer period than drinking a glass of apple juice, don't you think ?

The issue here is that the thyroid gland can only analyze the rate at which the sugar level increases, and not the source it came from. So in this case, after having drunk the glass of juice, it will analyze the rate at which the blood sugar level increases. The thyroid assumes that in order for it to increase this quickly, you must have consumed fifty apples, even if you only drank the equivalent of ten apples. What should not be forgotten here is that the speed of assimilation comes into play.

As the conductor of the orchestra, the thyroid gland then orders the pancreas to secrete insulin in order to restore the blood sugar level, considering its estimate that you have eaten fifty apples. Since this is not true and you only took in the equivalent of ten apples, the thyroid is mistaken, and consequently it orders the pancreas to secrete too much insulin. The result is that an excessive amount of sugar is absorbed by your cells in order to be converted into glycogen by the liver. Your blood sugar level will decrease to normal levels, and for a while you may feel tired. The thyroid then notices that blood sugar has dropped below normal. It will then order the pancreas to secrete glucagon, the secretion of which permits the liver to take stored glycogen and convert it back into sugar to stabilize the blood sugar level to normal. The liver is considered the body's laboratory. It has various functions, including managing fat levels and blood quality.

While there is nothing wrong with drinking fruit juice, it is preferable to eat the whole fruit rather than just its juice. Our organism is built this way. Moderation is an important asset. Refined sugars such as those in candy and desserts may actually decrease your energy level rather than increasing it, as described above. Balance is important; a healthy and well-balanced body will not suffer from occasional abuse. But health problems may develop with repeated excesses.

Many children have concentration problems at school. These problems are often related to nutrition. When you consume refined or concentrated sugar, you constantly require the intervention of the pancreas and the liver. Once this pattern is developed, the thyroid can become overly excitable. What I mean to say is that with a diet rich in refined or concentrated sugar, the glandular system is solicited too often and develops a habit. Over time, even if you start to eat normally later on, the thyroid may order the pancreas to secrete too much insulin. It will react excessively, putting you in a state of low blood sugar, which leads to fatigue and possibly lack of concentration. Many people learn to live with such a state, believing that it is normal to feel tired, and they stop looking for reasons to explain their fatigue. Others will consume all kind of products like vitamins to try to function normally.

Sooner or later, because it is secreting insulin to excess, the pancreas may stop functioning normally. This may be the beginning of diabetes. When they were younger, many of today's diabetics had hypoglycemia. If they had known back then about their low blood sugar and its cause, they would probably have corrected the problem with a proper diet and would live normally today without diabetes.

The liver, provided with nutrition rich in sugar and fat, is called on to excess. Like the pancreas it can become diseased, and many different health problems can develop.

I don't want to go into too many details about blood sugar here. It is a very interesting subject that is covered in various books. I just want you to realize the importance of a good diet in performing physical activities or simply living a healthy life, and to make you aware of the fact that yes, our diet can give us energy, and after a meal we can feel energetic and not necessarily sleepy.

Our bodies are complex, and they have certain peculiarities that we must respect. This will be explained more clearly in the chapter on "Nutritional Combinations."

COMPLEX SUGARS

Grains, vegetables, and flour all contain complex sugars that we call starch and dextrin.

> **Important:** complex sugars are absorbed relatively slowly, making them an excellent choice that interferes less with our blood sugar levels.

LIPIDS

Lipid molecules consist of carbon, hydrogen, and oxygen.

- Essential fatty acids are part of this group.
- Bile, secreted by the liver, emulsifies lipids into fine particles to allow enzymes to better digest them in the small intestine in the form of fatty acids and glycerol.

FATTY ACIDS

There are four main fatty acids:

- **Saturated**
- **Trans**
- **Monounsaturated**
- **Polyunsaturated**

SATURATED FATTY ACIDS

- Found mainly in animal products
- Solid at room temperature
- Polyunsaturated essential fatty acids are not supplied by these fat types.

A few sources: meat, poultry, butter, chocolate, cheese, milk, egg yolks, palm oil, coconut oil, and vegetable oil

TRANS FATS

- Found in small quantities in a natural state in certain foods: milk products, beef, and lamb

- Trans fatty acid is formed when a food manufacturer injects hydrogen into liquid oil to transform it into a semisolid fat such as shortening or margarine. This process extends the shelf life of the food containing these products and gives them a better appearance.

A few sources:

- Foods containing certain margarines, in particular hard margarine

- Foods fried in hydrogenated oil

- Bakery products (biscuits, cakes, croissants) made with shortening or hydrogenated fat or oil

MONOUNSATURATED AND POLYUNSATURATED FATTY ACIDS

- Found mainly in natural foods such as nuts and avocados

- Liquid at room temperature

- Essential fatty acids (polyunsaturated fatty acids) are present in this form of fat.

- Easily react with oxygen, light, and heat, and decompose rapidly; must be kept refrigerated

Sources of mono and polyunsaturated fatty acids:

- **Monounsaturated:** avocados, cashews, Peanuts, Peanut butter, Olives

- **Polyunsaturated:** safflower oil, sunflower oil, almonds, soy, canola oil

ROLE OF LIPIDS

- Constitute a good source of concentrated energy – twice that of carbohydrates and protein

- Transport and absorb fat-soluble vitamins A, D, E, and K

- Increase energy reserves, which are stored in the fat tissue

- Supply essential acids

- Insulate and protect organs like the liver, heart, and nerves

- Provide a sense of fullness by slowing stomach digestion

- Help maintain a constant body temperature

- Help nerve conduction and improve memory

ESSENTIAL ACIDS

- Help to obtain healthy skin

- Decrease blood cholesterol levels

- Act at the level of cellular membrane permeability

- Should be consumed in moderation because in excess they may become harmful

Sources: safflower, sunflower, sesame, flax, soy beans, corn. Consume only cold-pressed oils, and store these oils protected from light and heat.

Requirements: 1 tablespoon per day of cold-pressed oil or ¼ cup of seeds

EFFECTS OF FAT ON HEALTH

Polyunsaturated and monounsaturated fatty acids tend to decrease the risk of heart disease. It is therefore healthy to include them in our diet. On the contrary, saturated and trans fatty acids are damaging to our health. They tend to increase the risk of heart disease. According to studies, saturated fat increases our good cholesterol (HDL) level, but at the same time, they increase our bad cholesterol (LDL) level. Trans fat increases LDL levels. LDL is a known risk factor for heart disease. It also decreases HDL levels. HDL protects us against heart disease.

> **Note:** the body can produce certain fatty acids when needed. There are three polyunsaturated fatty acids that it cannot produce. They are linoleic acid, linolenic acid, and arachidonic acid. We have to provide our bodies with an appropriate supply of these through food.

PROTEINS

- Proteins are molecules composed of amino acids.

- They are digested at first in the stomach and later in the small intestine, where they are absorbed in the form of amino acids.

ROLE

Proteins serve in the construction, maintenance, and repair of cells as well as hair and nails, flexible skin, muscle fibers, bones, internal organs, the brain, injured tissue, hormones, and more.

Sources of Protein and Proportion of Protein They Contain

Vegetable origin:		Animal origin:	
Legumes	30%	Cheese	24%
Nuts and seeds	15%	Roast Beef	24%
Cereals	15%	Other meat	20%
Bread	7%	Fish	16%
		Eggs	13%

THE EIGHT ESSENTIAL AMINO ACIDS

- Isoleucine
- Phenylalanine
- Leucine
- Threonine
- Lysine
- Tryptophan
- Methionine
- Valine

Vegetable protein can be deficient in some essential amino acids. This deficiency prevents our bodies from using the protein completely. When there is an insufficient quantity of an essential amino acid, it decreases the quality of the protein. If you consume food that contains 100 percent of seven of the eight essential amino acids but only 10 percent of the eight, the body will only use 10 percent of the total protein in the food.

In order to obtain our principal proteins from vegetable sources, we have to combine foods that contain limited amino acids to allow maximum utilization of all proteins.

Proteins in Foods

Food	Rich in	Poor in
Legumes	Lysine Methionine	Tryptophan
Nuts and seeds	Tryptophan	Lysine
Cereals	Tryptophan Methionine	Lysine
Dairy products	Lysine	

With this table, we understand why:

Cereals + legumes = complete protein

Legumes + nuts and seeds = complete protein

Milk products + cereals = complete protein

There are other possible combinations: eggs and dairy products, being of animal origin, are complete proteins. When consumed with a vegetable protein, they adequately provide full protein. Green vegetables with cereals offer also complete protein. Therefore, eat lots of green vegetables with your pasta.

Notes

- The body does not have a protein reserve. This is why our daily food intake must contain protein.

- Animal protein is complete because it contains all the essential amino acids.

- To be complete, a protein must possess the eight essential amino acids in the right proportions.

We have already seen that the human digestive system is very complex. The different substances secreted by the mouth, the stomach, and the intestines must digest nutrients by absorbing them correctly to nourish all our tissues.

Depending of the type of food consumed, the glands must first recognize the nutrients and then secrete the specific digestive juice necessary for their absorption.

Carbohydrates (starches and sugars) are digested first in the mouth in a pH-neutral environment through the secretion of the ptyalin enzyme. Later, they are digested in the intestines in an alkaline environment by other amylase enzymes. The protease enzyme, secreted by the stomach glands, breaks down proteins into polypeptides.

Since carbohydrates are mostly not transformed in the stomach, their passage through this organ must be rapid. If they are consumed with proteins, they will stay in the stomach while the proteins are transformed into amino acids. The hydrochloric acid necessary for this protein digestion can considerably reduce the nutritional value of food containing carbohydrates. This mix favors fermentation and can produce elements that are harmful to our health. This is why nutritional combinations are very useful.

People with good digestion may not feel digestive discomfort. Occasional bad nutritional combinations are basically acceptable. But if you have poor nutrition with incompatible nutritional combinations for long periods of time, you may overwork your digestive system. After many years of such behavior, you may experience certain disorders in various body systems. Certain foods that are not completely digested may become a kind of toxin for the body and are therefore detrimental to our health in general.

The main goal of good nutritional combinations is to favor the complete digestion of nutrients as follows

>   **Proteins = polypeptides = amino acids**
>
>   **Lipids = fatty acids and glycerol**
>
>   **Carbohydrates = maltose = glucose**
>
>   **Maltose = glucose**
>
>   **Sucrose = fructose and glucose**

Cells in the intestines accept food in the form of amino acids, fatty acids, glycerol, glucose, fructose, and galactose. When you eat a meal that respects good nutritional combinations, nutrient absorption occurs easily without producing harmful effects on your health.

The following are a few points on good nutritional combinations.

1. A FRUIT MEAL

Fruit is very nutritious, but since its sugars are mainly in the form of fructose, it is digested very rapidly. Therefore it is preferable to not consume it with starches and proteins, which need more time to digest.

Morning is when our sugar needs are the greatest. Fruit is perfectly suited to a morning meal.

2. SEMIACIDIC FRUITS WITH ACIDIC OR MILD FRUITS

Semiacidic fruits can be consumed at the same time as acidic fruits or mild fruits.

3. MILD AND ACIDIC FRUITS

Mild fruits require more digestion time than acidic fruits. It is not recommended to consume them at the same meal.

4. NEUTRAL FRUITS

Neutral fruits digest better when consumed alone. Example of neutral fruits are melons, cantaloupes, and watermelon. They can be part of the same meal.

5. GREEN VEGETABLES WITH STARCHES

This combination is recommended because it favors nutrient absorption. The body tolerates consuming raw green vegetables with oil. One quirk about starches: since food acids inhibit secretion of ptyalin, the essential enzyme for digesting starch in the mouth, acidic foods like tomatoes should not be consumed during a starch meal. Starch meals are recommended for noon.

6. ONE STARCH AT A TIME

More than one starch should not be consumed at the same meal. When one starch is accompanied by raw or slightly steamed vegetables, digestion is greatly improved.

7. GREEN VEGETABLES AND PROTEIN

Minerals and vitamins supplied by raw vegetables facilitate digestion of fatty proteins like nuts and cheese. Because the structure of protein is different in each food, it is not a good idea to have a meal composed of more than one source of protein per day. Protein should be accompanied by green vegetables, preferably raw.

Since proteins help to stabilize blood sugar, it is a good idea to consume them during an evening meal, which will help stabilize blood sugar during sleep.

8. PROTEIN WITH STARCHES AND FATS

Since protein is digested in an acidic environment and starches are digested in an alkaline environment, the combination of these two types of food during the same meal considerably impedes digestion. Fats decrease gastric secretions, so to ensure digestion is not delayed, we must avoid mixing fats and proteins.

Proper nutritional combinations are very important to reduce the energy required for digestion. Within our current modern lifestyles it is difficult to follow these recommendations all the time. When you are recovering from an illness or when you feel exhausted, fatigued, or overworked, you may find that your health benefits from these recommendations.

An athlete who wants to reach maximum energy potential must respect these proper nutritional combinations, which are complementary to training. If it is too difficult to follow all of these rules, at least attempt some of them. It is better to get as close as possible to following them than not to try to change at all. Here is a way to get close enough without too much difficulty.

It is relatively easy to respect the combinations of a fruit meal in the morning, a carbohydrate meal at noon, and one protein in the evening. Pay careful attention to proportions. For example, we know that the evening meal should be protein. If it is important for you to consume potatoes with your meal, your plate should contain a large proportion of proteins. If your plate contains a combination of ninety percent protein and ten percent starch (the potatoes), then digestion should perform relatively well. But if you consume protein and starch in equal amounts, digestion will be more difficult. Hydrochloric acid is secreted in the lower region of the stomach. Therefore it is not recommended that you eat the potatoes at the same time as the meat. If you start your meal by eating the meat first, it will make its way to the lower part of the stomach, where hydrochloric acid is mainly secreted. Potatoes eaten later will find themselves in the upper part of the stomach, less exposed to the acid during digestion.

We can apply the same principle in the morning, when the majority of the meal should be composed of fruit, and at noon, when it should be mainly composed of carbohydrates.

If desserts are too hard to eliminate from your diet, a small portion can be consumed at the noon meal and eliminated from the evening meal. As discussed previously, even if the combination on your plate is not perfect, your digestion will be easier if you observe these points.

WATER

Water is a source of life. The male body is approximately 70 percent water, and the female body is about 62 percent water. To meet its needs, the body must be supplied with half a gallon of water per day.

FUNCTION

1. Water is part of our tissues and bodily fluids : blood, lymph, and secretions.

2. Through perspiration and respiration, water helps to regulate body temperature.

3. Water is essential to transport nutrients to cells.

4. Cells use water to eliminate waste.

5. Water aids in the elimination of waste through the kidneys, skin, lungs, and intestines.

Notes

• We must refrain from drinking for at least fifteen minutes before a meal and wait at least two hours afterward.

• It is preferable to drink water at room temperature and for its consumption to be equally distributed through the day; this means six to eight glasses of water per day, beginning when we get out of bed in the morning, before and after meals, and during the evening, up to approximately two hours before bed.

Appendix

EXPLANATION OF THE FORMULA $f = M \times V$

The formula is derived from the formula p = mv, where **p** represents momentum (kinetic impetus), **m** is the mass, and **v** is the speed. You might not be familiar with the term *momentum*. What taekwondo practitioners want is to have powerful impact force. The force of impact is determined by the time the projected mass takes to change speed after a collision. Therefore, we cannot talk about impact force without being able to determine the target's capacity to change the speed of the projected mass in a certain time. The longer the time that the target is able to decrease the speed of the projected mass, the weaker the force of impact will be. It is also true that the more the target resists the change, the more rapidly the speed of the projected mass will decrease, and therefore the force of the impact will be greater.

If you cannot determine what the force of the movement's impact will be, you may decide what its momentum will be. What the target receives on impact is the momentum that has developed. The necessary time to decrease the speed of the movement will determine the force of the impact. No matter how well you succeed in developing the speed of the mass, the target will only receive the momentum. This momentum is the **p** obtained by multiplying the mass, **m**, by its speed, **v.**

In order to facilitate explanations in this book, instead of talking abut momentum, I have used the term **striking force,** which is more visual for most people. In order to respect the original formula, **p = mv,** I've used **f = mv.**

A few important notes:

• **When two masses come into collision in an isolated system,** meaning a system where no exterior forces interact with these masses, the sum of the quantity of movement that they possessed before the collision is the same after the collision. The quantity of movement that one mass will lose after a collision is therefore transferred to the other.

• **When one mass is moving,** meaning when one mass is displaced at a certain speed, momentum results. When this

**A few formulas that helped me develop
the hip-propulsion movement:**

1. $p = mv$, where p is momentum, m is the mass, and v is the speed. Kinetic momentum always goes in the same direction as the speed.

2. $\triangle p = m\triangle v$, where $\triangle p$ represents the change in momentum, m is the mass, and $\triangle v$ is the change in speed

3. $f = ma$, where f is the force, m is the mass, and a is acceleration

4. $a = \triangle v \div t$: If $f = ma$, we can say that $f = m\triangle v \div t$. It is then true to say that $ft = m\triangle v$.

5. By definition, we know that the impetus is the applied force multiplied by time: $impetus = ft = m\triangle v$ = change in momentum.

6. $impetus = \triangle p$ = change in momentum

mass in movement collides with another mass, force is developed if the moving mass changes speed. The time this mass takes to change its speed will determine the force of impact. For example, imagine a car moving at a speed of sixty miles per hour. The speed multiplied by the car's mass is its momentum. To stop the car, an exterior force must be applied to it. The larger the force, the more rapidly the car will slow.

Conclusion

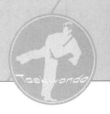

"Without the rocks, the waves would never get so high."[1]
I love this sentence because it shows us that obstacles can
help us to grow. Often, it is our attitude that makes the
difference. We want to be physically strong, so we engage
in physical activity. But what happens to the mental side?

Self-defense and sparring as taught by taekwondo make interesting
practice. But when we grant importance to every detail in order to
achieve maximum force using minimum energy in a precise technique
delivered with precise timing, we see a degree of self-awareness in
every technique, and a route is revealed that becomes more and
more accessible. That route, without limits, becomes our path. By
presenting my ideas in this book, I wanted to provide precise details
that will allow you to use taekwondo as a tool to guide you on that
route. The nutritional advice will help you naturally obtain maximum
performance from your body. The section on reflexology in this
book simplifies certain techniques from that science to enable its
easy use. And though it is a reference guide for high-performance
athletes, this book also contains elements suitable for taekwondo
practitioners of all levels.

1   Roger Nimier, *Le Hussard Bleu* (Paris: Gallimard, 1950).

Remember : Perfection does not exist. If you believe that you have reached perfection, then you have ceased to evolve. Your learning resides in the attitude that you adopt.

I will conclude with a short story I wrote about appearances.

Good luck !

– Master Gilles R. Savoie

APPEARANCES

Winter is finally over, and the wind has died down. Gloves, hats, and scarves can be put away, and we can leave our cocoon. Spring prepares us for the summer's heat and bright colors. Spring's yellow, red, and white flowers and birdsong attract us outside to get a little bit of sun.

I walk on a sandy beach with my wife and children. The sun's reflection on the waves extraordinarily enhances the outside colors. The sounds follow a rhythm so predicable that we can let ourselves dance under the soft music of the seagulls' songs.

Suddenly I lose my footing. What happened ? A wave pulled out the sand that was supporting my feet and unbalanced me. I open my eyes and my surroundings look different. My children are smiling. I stand up with difficulty to regain my balance. Everything looks unstable. Looking at my wife playing with the kids, as if she were one of them, I realize that they are all barefoot. Is that the solution to their balance ? If I dare remove my shoes and socks, to better feel the sand under my bare feet, will I recover my balance ? No, I don't want to try that. I might catch cold and get sick. The sky is getting gray. Another question arises … will it rain ? My umbrella will protect me. I open it, just in case.

During that time, my kids are looking towards the sea, astounded, smiling with their eyes, barefoot in the tiny grains that sparkle like crystal. They are building sand castles with the help of their mother. From a child's point of view, time seems like an eternity, and they take advantage of every moment. So little is required to make their eyes sparkle like stars. A little attention from us, a little love, and their world changes. Only the present exists for them, since tomorrow seems too far and yesterday is already forgotten. Although we don't actually know it, this love in the present has great influence on their appearance tomorrow.

When I return to my memories I always see the beach on a sunny day, with soft warm sand under a sky so blue that clouds dare not appear. I run on the sandy beach, not falling, changing direction at will. The waves caress my feet as they clean the sand.

Today, things have changed. The wave under my feet has retreated to the sea, making me lose my balance. Its gray color has given it so much energy that it has hit me with a sly violence. How could I have anticipated this? What do my children see that I don't? The sky is gray; the sea is taking on its reflection. The sea is not very welcoming. I can't tell if it will rain or not. If it were going to rain, I would have stayed home, where I was sheltered. If the sky were blue, I would take advantage of the sun. But no, the sky is gray. Will it rain or not? I am relatively safe with my umbrella. The problem is that it stops me from seeing the horizon. Is that important? I am here on the beach. Why do I need to see the horizon with this gray sky?

Why don't my children ask themselves these questions? Have they no fear of falling, of catching cold, of getting wet as they run like that on the sand, where millions of tiny sand grains roll under their feet?

In the gray, there is black and white. Maybe my kids see the white in the gray, and I on the other hand see only the black. Therefore, is everything illusory? Is what I see in reality only an interpretation of my emotions? Where do these feelings come from? And if my umbrella is only an illusion, if it rains, I will get wet.

The sand slides under my feet, and I try with all my strength to stabilize myself, not to fall. My children play, fall, get up, and will even have more fun if it rains. But what do they see that I don't? How can my wife play with them as if she were their age?

Finally, I decide to dare to do it. I take off my shoes and socks. Maybe my bare feet on the sand will change the appearance of things in my eyes. What do I have to lose? The freedom of my children helps me overcome my fears, and I put my bare feet in those millions of grains of sand that might scratch my skin. Surprisingly, they are not as cold as I though they would be, and those little crystals actually tickle my skin with an overwhelming gentleness rather than scratching. The waves continue to remove the sand from beneath my feet. I feel it sliding, and I can easily get my balance before losing it. Is this the solution? I was mistaken, thinking all those years that I was balanced. To walk, I have to put myself in imbalance! In reality, imbalance allows me to walk. But if I don't want to turn in circles and get lost, I have to feel where my imbalance projects me so that I can orient my body toward the desired direction. It is then by acquiring my balance that I can walk.

The waves in time change the beach's appearance. By confronting it, in good or bad weather, they have changed it. Yet they slide well over each other. They have modified their form, one to the other, in a way that they are still here today. They have adapted. Evolution is therefore adaptation to change. Change causes imbalance, and the quest to regain balance allows walking.

I have to see things through my kids' eyes. Since the outer world is illusory, my emotions must be as close as possible to the heart of the child within me, the one that has not been spoiled by bitterness and hypocrisy. Fear of the unknown and fear of change erect barriers that hold us down. Children are not scared of tomorrow. For them, tomorrow does not exist. They live fully today. Why put so much energy and attention into something that does not even exist?

This child in me still exists. For many years I have dressed him in many different feelings, so when I look in a mirror I don't recognize him anymore. The mirror, still, is just an illusion.

My son turns toward me, happy to see my bare feet in the sand. Suddenly, in his eyes, I see the child in myself. I feel his joy, his love, his sincerity, free from all the feelings that suffocate him. This emotion sends a warm tingling that pervades my whole body. Arms surround me, and I feel the softness of my wife's cheek on mine. She notices that something has happened to me. With her gaze, an intense communication starts. No words are sufficient to express it, but she understands. Words are useless, and images are illusory. What is left? Is it love?

Love is an emotion, but for it to be intense it must be expressed with sincerity. Otherwise, different illusions take form, preventing us from feeling its full power and seeing where the direction of balance is heading – our lives. If we lose this sense, we turn in circles with no destination and then fall.

Evolution is adaptation to change, and change causes imbalance. Since the quest to achieve balance allows us to walk, and thus to go to a desired destination, I need to see through the eyes of the child in me: does illusion exist to allow evolution?

Acknowledgments

I would like to thank my students.
With all of their questions they have been
excellent teachers for me.

To my parents, Norbert and Alice,
in the hope that I have become what they expected.

To Simone,
an inspiration for the joy in my life.

To my children, François and Jérémi,
a little of my story is for you.

And thanks to my wife, Nicole,
my North Star.

About the Author

Gilles R. Savoie was born in Campbellton, New Brunswick, and began his martial arts training in 1969, at the age of nine. He first became a black belt in karate and jujitsu (an art primarily based on self-defense). Sparring with other martial artists introduced him to taekwondo, which at the time was not a very popular martial art in Canada. The power and speed of taekwondo impressed him so much that he decided to deepen his knowledge of this art.

In 1981 he began to study under Master Chong Lee, who had brought the discipline to Canada in 1964 and had trained some of the best Canadian champions. After intense effort and disciplined training, Savoie was promoted to black belt. Today he is a taekwondo master with a seventh-dan black belt.

Savoie has also studied phytotherapy (a form of natural medicine) and reflexology (therapeutic massage of reflex points), which he continues to practice. Master Savoie frequently gives seminars and presentations on the biomechanics of taekwondo. He is currently the technical director of the taekwondo association in the Gaspe region of Québec, Canada, where he lives.